High-Yield Microbiology and Infectious Diseases

High-Yield Microbiology and Infectious Diseases

Louise B. Hawley, Ph.D.

Assistant Professor of Microbiology

Department of Medical Microbiology and Immunology

UMD School of Medicine

University of Minnesota, Duluth

Duluth, Minnesota

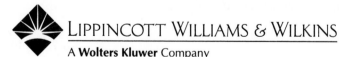

LIPPINCOTT WILLIAMS & WILKINS

A **Wolters Kluwer** Company

Philadelphia · Baltimore · New York · London
Buenos Aires · Hong Kong · Sydney · Tokyo

Editor: Elizabeth A. Nieginski
Editorial Director: Julie P. Martinez
Development Editors: Rachel A. Bedard and Rosanne Hallowell
Managing Editors: Marette D. Magargle-Smith and Karla Schroeder
Marketing Manager: Aimee Sirmon
Illustrator: Wayne E. Heim

351 West Camden Street
Baltimore, Maryland 21201–2436 USA

530 Walnut Street
Philadelphia, Pennsylvania 19106 USA

Printed in the United States of America

The publishers have made every effort to trace the copyright holders for borrowed material. If they have inadvertently overlooked any, they will be pleased to make the necessary arrangements at the first opportunity.

To purchase additional copies of this book call our customer service department at **(800) 638-3030** or fax orders to **(301) 824-7390**. International customers should call **(301) 714-2324**.

02
3 4 5 6 7 8 9 10

Dedication

To my wonderful, supportive, and tolerant husband and daughters, and to my mother, who gave me many essential early lessons on teaching

Contents

V. PARASITES

VI. INFECTIOUS DISEASES

Preface

High-Yield™ Microbiology and Infectious Diseases provides a review of these subject areas as they have typically been covered on Step 1 of the United States Medical Licensing Examination (USMLE) and Comprehensive Osteopathic Medical Licensing Examination (COMLEX). I have also included topics that I anticipate will be added to the exams this year.

The material is presented using four different approaches:

1. **Bug Parade Approach: Microbiology, Bacteria, Viruses, Fungi, Parasites (Chapters 1–34).** These chapters cover major microbial and parasitic genera and species, presenting important organism characteristics and the diseases each organism causes. There are separate chapters covering bacterial and viral genetics; bacterial genetic concepts are generously illustrated.

2. **Organ-System/Disease Approach: Infectious Diseases (Chapters 35–43).** Pneumonias, rashes, and other diseases and conditions are presented in an easy-to-use clinical vignette format suitable for both fast review and self-testing. Each "high-yield" case is followed by the questions that are most likely to be asked on the exam. You won't have to flip pages for the answers—they're right below the questions! (For self-testing, use a cover sheet to cover the answers.)

3. **Comparative Microbiology Approach (Chapter 44).** The comparative chapter groups microorganisms according to important features—for example, "Antiphagocytic Structures," or "Toxins with ADP-Ribosyl Transferase Activity." The outline format allows you to either quickly scan for review or test yourself (using a cover sheet) to ensure that, when these features are used as clues on the exam, you will answer the questions with ease. This section also includes tables that highlight important toxins, culture media, and modes of transmission important in differentiating infectious disease agents.

4. **High-Yield Case Set-up Approach.** This section consists of high-yield case set-ups, which are cases composed of essential clues without the easily changeable "window dressing." The case set-ups are presented in random order; each case is followed by a series of likely exam questions, with answers immediately following the questions. The format allows for both quick review and self-testing. Much faster and broader self-testing is possible with this format than with multiple-choice questions.

The inclusion of these four different approaches gives you several options. For example, you can focus on a "bug" approach if you were taught according to an "organ-system" approach—or vice versa. Or you can study the entire book, which will provide the repetition you will need to retain the many facts crucial to analyzing the exam's clinical cases and answering the questions.

Other features that are used throughout the book to enhance your review include illustrations, tables, boldface terms, and **memory tricks** (identified with the symbol ◑). Organisms that are particularly likely to be on the exam are often identified simply as "high-yield." In conjunction with the *High-Yield™* series outline format, these features provide for an efficient review.

The USMLE's (and COMLEX's) Strategy For Microbiology Testing

On the USMLE and COMLEX examinations, many questions start with a clinical scenario. For the microbiology and infectious disease questions, you will need to recognize the disease presentation and identify the causative agent based on clinical or basic science information. You may be asked to identify the causative agent, but more frequently that question will be skipped and instead you will be asked a basic science question about the causative agent, the disease, or therapeutic mechanisms. For instance, the exam may present a case history of a child with cough, coryza, conjunctivitis, and small gray oral lesions with a red base, which is followed by the development of a macular papular rash from the ears down that becomes confluent on the face. You might be asked to identify the family of the viral causative agent (measles is caused by Rubeola which is a Paramyxovirus), or the replicative intermediate of the causative agent (it replicates through a positive RNA intermediate). In infections where there is a dominant causative agent (e.g., a urinary tract infection), you will need to know what it is (*E. coli*). In some cases, distinguishing clues will be used to point you to a specific but less common organism; for example, if a catalase-positive, Gram-positive coccus is the predominant organism in a urinary tract infection, then the infecting organism is *Staphylococcus saprophyticus*. Clues may include bug characteristics, virulence factors, geography, route and timing of exposure, patient's age, underlying condition, and symptomology.

There will also be questions comparing different organisms or groups of organisms, toxins or other virulence factors. *Example:* A case of pneumonia (maybe without geographical or environmental clues!) with a description of the causative agent in tissue, such as "broad-based budding yeast in tissue which grows as a filamentous form with nondescript small conidia at room temperature" (*Blastomyces dermatitidis*). The next question might be about the disease's endemic regions (great riverbeds in U.S. and the southeastern U.S. seaboard states), or where in the environment the exposure originated (high-organic soil with rotting wood). [An association with bats would indicate *Histoplasma*; with pigeons, *Cryptococcus*; and with desert sand, *Coccidioides*.] Because of the low computer screen resolution on the computerized exams, microscopic images are less likely to be used than verbal descriptions.

In the great majority of questions, high-order thinking will be required—you will have to piece together several clues. This book presents the essential database of concepts and facts that will enable you to answer the questions. The fourfold approach of *High-Yield™ Microbiology and Infectious Diseases* not only provides the repetition needed to improve retention of the data, but also provides several options for optimizing your review. In addition, the Infectious Disease section and the High-Yield Cases in Chapter 45 will provide you some insight and practice into the problem solving.

If you have any comments about this High-Yield™ title or suggestions for the next edition, please send them to the publisher at Lippincott Williams & Wilkins, Review Books, Rose Tree Corporate Center, Building II, Suite 5025, 1400 N. Providence Road, Media, PA 19063-2043, or via e-mail to Rounds@lww.com.

I wish you good luck!

Louise B. Hawley, Ph.D.

Acknowledgments

Publication of a book is a team project! I want to send my thanks to *all* the talented staff of Lippin-cott, Williams & Wilkins. In particular, I want to thank:

Elizabeth Nieginski for her editorial vision;
Rachel Bedard and Rosanne Hallowell for their expert language crafting;
Wayne Heim for his masterful transformation of my lines and squiggles into useful illustrations;
Marette Magargle-Smith and Karla Schroeder for facilitating the production;
Aimee Simon for her marketing expertise.

I would also like to thank the compositor and printer, members of the team whom I have never met, who played critical roles in the publication of the book.

I
Microbiology

1

General Microbiology

I. **INTRODUCTION.** Each major microbial group has different characteristics that result in distinct disease mechanisms, varying host responses, and the need for different interventions.

II. **TWO CELL TYPES.** Of the cellular microorganisms, there are two different cell types: **prokaryotes** and **eukaryotes**.

   A. Animals (including **humans** and **animal parasites**), **plants**, and **fungi** are the major **eukaryotes**.

   B. Bacteria are the major **prokaryotes**.

   C. **Major differences** are outlined in **Table 1-1. Relative diameters** of microbial groups are shown in **Figure 1-1.**

III. **MICROBIAL GROUPS** are presented here from simplest to most complex, but in the remainder of the book microbial groups are presented in order of their frequency on the United States Medical Licensing Examination (USMLE) Step 1.

   A. Prions (PrP) are **noncellular infectious proteins.**

       1. Prions are associated with **subacute spongiform encephalopathies** like **Creutzfeldt-Jakob disease.**

       2. Prions are **naked proteins** that have the **same amino acid sequence as certain normal cellular proteins,** but are **folded differently.**

       3. The normal human cellular proteins (now referred to as **cellular prionlike proteins** or **PrP^c**) are coded for by cellular genes.

       4. Once prion proteins gain entry into the human cells, **they modify the folding of normal PrP^c, turn those proteins into additional prions,** and eventually cause neurologic degeneration.

   B. Viruses are **obligate intracellular organisms** (i.e., they cannot be grown outside a host cell).

       1. Viruses are composed of **either RNA *or* DNA** surrounded by various proteins. They may or may not have an envelope.

       2. Viruses are **noncellular.** They take over host cells and, using the viral nucleic acid, direct the synthesis and assembly of viral components to make new virus.

   C. Bacteria are prokaryotic cells.

       1. Bacteria have **70S ribosomes,** complex cell walls of **peptidoglycan** (except for mycoplasmas), and **no sterols** (except in *Mycoplasma* membranes).

Table 1-1
Prokaryotic vs Eukaryotic Cellular Organization

Characteristic	Prokaryotic Cells (Bacteria)	Eukaryotic Cells (Fungi, Plants, Protozoans, and Animals Including Humans)
Genetic organization	1 circular DNA molecule organized into multiple "loops" with nonhistone proteins and RNA	Linear DNA condensed with histones
	1 chromosome, multiple copies	More than one chromosome
	Mono- and polycistronic mRNA	Monocistronic mRNA
	Exons; no introns	Exons and introns
	No nuclear membrane	Nuclear membrane present
	Continuous DNA synthesis	G and S growth phases
Cytoplasmic structures	No mitochondria, no endoplasmic reticulum (ER), no lysosomes	Mitochondria, ER, ±lysosomes
	70S ribosomes (30S and 50S subunits)	80S ribosomes (40S and 60S subunits)
Nuclear/cell division	Binary fission (asexual)	Mitosis or meiosis with cytokinesis

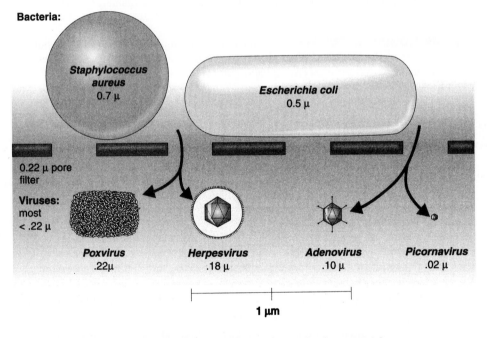

Bacteria:

Staphylococcus aureus 0.7 μ

Escherichia coli 0.5 μ

0.22 μ pore filter

Viruses: most < .22 μ

Poxvirus .22μ

Herpesvirus .18 μ

Adenovirus .10 μ

Picornavirus .02 μ

1 μm

By Contrast: Fungal hyphae 3μ (septate) up to 8 μ (non-septate)
Yeasts 3μ (*Histoplasma*) up to 20μ (*Cryptococcus*)
Red blood cells 7-8μ
Worm eggs 16-80μ
Worms 300μ and up

Figure 1-1.   Comparative diameters of microorganisms.

2. Bacteria **divide asexually by binary fission.**

D. **Fungi** are **eukaryotic organisms.**

    1. Fungi have complex carbohydrate cell walls containing **chitin,** glucans, and mannans.

    2. Fungal membranes have **ergosterol** as the major **sterol,** allowing treatment with **imidazoles and polyene drugs.**

    3. **Fungi** include the **yeasts, filamentous molds, dimorphic fungi, and mushrooms.**

E. **Parasites*** are eukaryotic cells. The animal parasites are the protozoans, worms, and insects that live on other organisms. These animals have sterols in their cell membranes but do not have cell walls.

---

*Note: The term parasite is used (1) specifically to mean the animal parasites such as protozoans and helminths and (2) more broadly to define an organism that derives its nutrition from another organism. In general in this text, the term "parasite" refers specifically to animal parasites, and "pathogen" will be substituted for the broader usage.

//
Bacteria

2

Bacterial Structure

I. CELL ENVELOPE. The cell envelope consists of the cytoplasmic membrane, cell wall, outer membrane (Gram-negative bacteria only), and, for some bacteria, capsule.

  A. Role of the cell envelope. In addition to protecting the bacterial cell, the cell envelope components play a major role in **adherence** to or invasion of human cells, **virulence,** and **stimulation of the immune response.**

  B. Structures, chemistry, and function

  1. The **components** of the cell envelope, as well as the **chemistry** and **functions** of these structures, differ between Gram-positive and Gram-negative bacteria, as depicted in **Figures 2-1 and 2-2.** (Note: This **high-yield information** is likely to be tested on the USMLE Step 1 exam.

  2. Differences in the cross-linkage of the peptidoglycan of Gram-positive and Gram-negative bacteria are shown in **Figure 2-3.** These differences lead to **differential retention of the Gram dye complex.**

  a. The **Gram-positive** peptidoglycan "net" with its many pentaglycine bridges is more tightly cross-linked, so it **retains the large dye complex** inside the peptidoglycan.

  b. The **Gram-negative** outer membrane is damaged by the organic solvent decolorizer. The thinner, less cross-linked peptidoglycan **does not retain the dye** in decolorization.

  c. Table 2-1 reviews the **Gram stain steps.**

  3. Differences between the cell envelopes of Gram-positive and Gram-negative bacteria are highlighted in **Table 2-2.**

II. SURFACE PROTRUSIONS

  A. Flagella (not found on all bacteria) are semi-rigid, helical filaments made up of protein. **Counterclockwise rotation** produces **directed motion; clockwise rotation** produces **tumbling.** A flagellum is shown in **Figure 2-4.**

  B. Fimbriae (pili) are proteinaceous microfilaments extending through the cell envelope and beyond. They may be categorized as **adhesins or lectins** (binding to specific host cell receptors), **evasins** (inhibiting phagocytic uptake in the nonimmune individual), or **sex pili** (establishing the cell-to-cell contact needed for bacterial **conjugation**).

  C. Envelope surface antigens are teichoic acids or certain outer membrane proteins (OMPs) that affect **adherence** or **virulence** (such as the ability to invade nonphagocytic host cells).

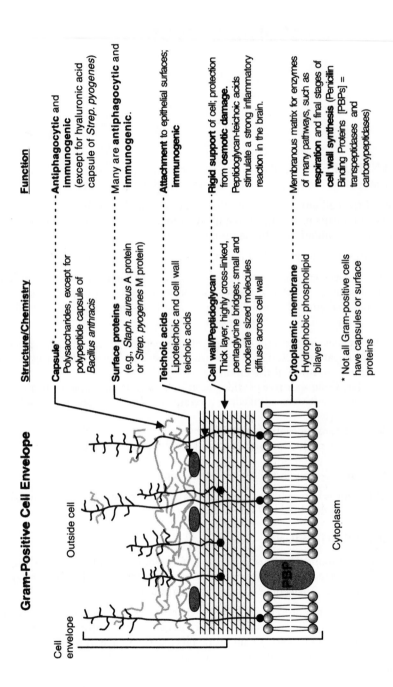

Figure 2-1.   Gram-positive cell envelope showing structures and describing their chemistry and function.

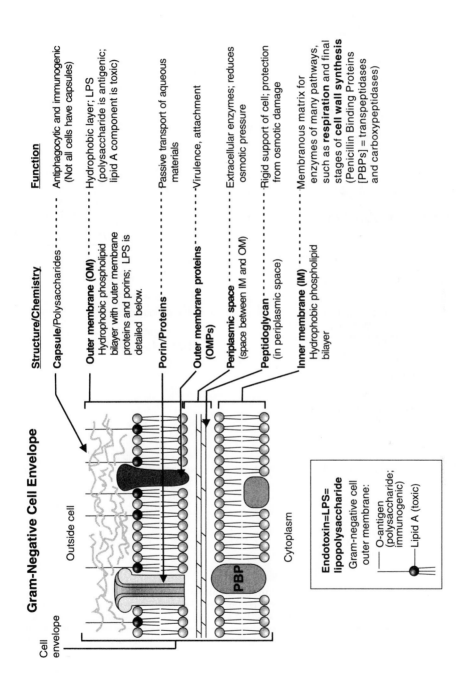

Figure 2-2. Gram-negative cell envelope showing structures and describing their chemistry and function.

Comparison of Peptidoglycan in Bacteria

Gram-Positive	**Gram-Negative**

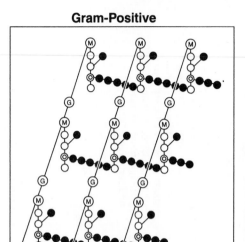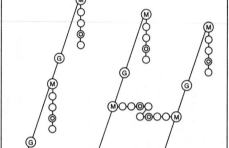

◎ = L-lysine or diaminopimelic acid, which is unique to bacterial peptidoglycan and not found in proteins

● = glycines making up penta-glycine bridge cross-linking (only in Gram-positives)

Ⓜ = N-acetylmuramic acid

Ⓖ = N-acetylglucosamine

○ = other amino acids

Gram-positive cells have up to 60 layers like this.

◎ = diaminopimelic acid

Ⓜ = N-acetylmuramic acid

Ⓖ = N-acetylglucosamine

○ = other amino acids

Gram-negative cells have 1 to 3 layers of peptidoglycan.

Figure 2-3.   Comparison of cross-linkage of peptidoglycan in Gram-positive and Gram-negative bacteria.

Table 2-1
Gram Stain Procedure

Step	Gram-positive cell	Gram-negative cell
1. Gram's crystal violet (a small dye particle)	Dark purple (small dye particle)	Dark purple (small dye particle)
2. Gram's iodine (a complexing agent or mordant)	Dark purple (large dye complex)	Dark purple (large dye complex)
3. Acetone alcohol decolorization	Purple	Colorless
4. Safranin counterstain (a pale red dye)	Purple/blue	Red/pink

Table 2-2
Gram-Positive vs Gram-Negative Bacteria: Comparison of Cell Envelope Features

	Gram-Positive Bacteria	**Gram-Negative Bacteria**
Envelope layers	Two layers: **1.** Peptidoglycan (open, netlike) **2.** Cytoplasmic membrane (hydrophobic) Resistant to antibody and complement-mediated killing, but susceptible to lysozyme	Three layers: **1.** Outer membrane or OM (hydrophobic) **2.** Peptidoglycan (open, netlike) **3.** Inner membrane (hydrophobic) OM reduces susceptibility to lysozyme but is susceptible to damage by antibody and complement
Unique features	Teichoic acids	Outer membrane and endotoxin* Periplasmic space (between membranes) Porins[†]
Methods of attachment to human cells	Teichoic acids *Streptococcus pyogenes:* also pili (M protein) Specific virulence factors	Pili Specific virulence factors
Surface antigens	Teichoic acids Surface-specific proteins, for example: • M protein: Group A *Streptococcus* (fimbria) • Tuberculin: *Mycobacterium tuberculosis* • A protein: *Staphylococcus aureus* Capsular material (except *Streptococcus pyogenes* hyaluronic acid capsule) Flagella Other colonizing/virulence factors	O antigens (polysaccharide of LPS) Outer membrane proteins Fimbria and pili Capsular material Flagella Other colonizing/virulence factors
Peptidoglycan (netlike, not hydrophobic)	Thick layer, highly cross-linked by pentaglycine bridges	Thin layer, not highly cross-linked
Effect of beta-lactam drugs	Antibiotic can diffuse directly through peptidoglycan and bind to penicillin-binding proteins, inhibiting cell wall cross-linkage. Gram-positive bacteria are generally more susceptible to beta-lactam drugs.	All antibiotics must penetrate porins. Some, like vancomycin, cannot. *Pseudomonas* is missing high-affinity porins. Periplasmic space allows accumulation of beta lactamases (if produced). Gram-negative bacteria are generally less susceptible. Beta-lactams are drugs of choice for some Gram-negative bacteria, such as *T. pallidum.*
Major triggers of inflammation	Peptidoglycan-teichoic acid	Endotoxin

*Listeria, which is Gram-positive, has a small amount of an endotoxin-like compound—ignore.
[†]Porins are also found in the mycobacteria spanning the waxy cell wall. Mycobacteria are Gram-positive and so do not have an outer membrane.

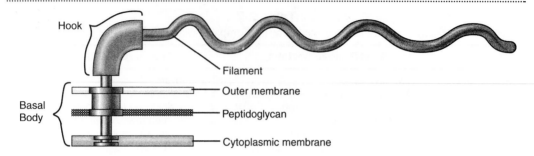

Figure 2-4.   Structure of a bacterial flagellum. (The one shown is a Gram-negative bacterium.)

    D. **Capsules** are **polysaccharides** that inhibit phagocytic uptake by a variety of mechanisms in nonimmune individuals.

III. INTERIOR STRUCTURES

    A. **Granules.** Bacteria polymerize and store compounds (like phosphates) that are required in large amounts. This reduces the osmotic pressure on the bacterial cell and may result in granules in the cells.

    B. **Lack of membrane-bound organelles.** Bacteria are prokaryotic and lack membrane-bound organelles (e.g., mitochondria and lysosomes). Respiratory enzymes and cytochromes are embedded in the cytoplasmic membrane.

    C. **Endospores.** Endospores occur in two Gram-positive genera of bacteria: *Bacillus* (aerobic) and *Clostridium* (anaerobic). Endospores **are resistant to killing** by boiling, cold, desiccation, and antiseptics. **Figure 2-5** describes sporulation and the structure of the endospore.

    D. **Chromosomes.** The **bacterial chromosome** is a **single,** covalently closed **circle of double-stranded DNA.** There may be multiple copies of the one chromosome.

Sporulating Genera: *Clostridium* and *Bacillus*

Function: Survival in adverse conditions (heat, chemicals, dessication, etc.)
No increase in cell numbers

Process:

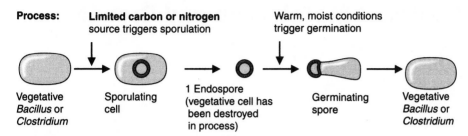

Mechanism of resistance:
Dehydration stabilizes proteins and nucleic acids.
Calcium dipicolinate is produced by sporulating cells and plays a role in dehydration of nucleic acid.
Calcium dipicolinate is unique to *Bacillus* and *Clostridium*.
Some new heat-resistant enzymes are produced.
Keratin coat provides protection.

Structure:

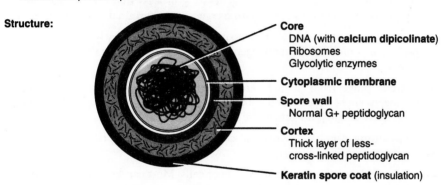

Figure 2-5. Sporulating process and the structure of an endospore. Sporulating genera are *Clostridium* or *Bacillus*.

3

Bacterial Metabolism and Growth

I. BACTERIAL METABOLISM

A. Pathogenic bacteria are **heterotrophs** (they derive their **energy from organic carbon** sources).

B. Organic compounds are broken down by **aerobic respiration** or **fermentation.**

1. **Aerobic respiration is an energy-generating process** that cycles sugars through glycolysis and the Krebs cycle, **with oxygen as the terminal electron acceptor.**

2. **Fermentation, an anaerobic process,** is the release of energy by metabolism of organic compounds using an endogenous organic compound as their terminal electron acceptor.

3. Bacteria **range from obligate anaerobes to obligate aerobes.** The majority of pathogens are facultative anaerobes that can metabolize aerobically depending on conditions. **High-yield genera** are listed in **Table 3-1.**

C. **Disease-causing bacteria** use organic compounds from living tissue and are called **pathogens** or **parasites.**

1. **Extracellular pathogens** grow outside of cells. Most can be routinely cultured in the laboratory on inert media. (Exception: *Treponema pallidum* cannot be cultured, so it is considered an obligate parasite.)

2. **Facultative intracellular pathogens** generally are found inside cells in the body, but can be grown in the laboratory.

3. **Obligate intracellular pathogens** grow only inside cells and cannot be cultured *in vitro* (e.g., *Mycobacterium leprae*, chlamydiae, and mycoplasmas).

D. Some nonpathogenic bacteria (called **commensals**) can live in or on people without causing significant disease. **Long-term commensals of the human body** are often referred to as **normal flora.**

II. BACTERIAL GROWTH is a coordinated process of increase in individual cell mass and size, followed by duplication of the chromosome and cell division.

A. Since **bacterial reproduction** involves duplication of DNA without the addition of outside DNA, bacterial cell division **is asexual** and gives rise to **genetically identical cells.** This process is called **binary fission,** because **one cell always gives rise to two cells (Figure 3-1A).**

B. Bacterial growth is **measured by two basic methods:**

Table 3-1
Aerobes and Anaerobes

Type of Organism	Definition	High-Yield Examples
Anaerobes	**Utilize fermentative pathways.** Most anaerobes **lack superoxide dismutase and catalase.** • **Obligate** anaerobes have only fermentative pathways and are killed by oxygen. • **Aerotolerant** anaerobes have no aerobic pathways but can **tolerate oxygen.**	*Actinomyces* *Bacteroides* *Clostridium**
Facultative anaerobes	Have **both aerobic respiration and fermentation** (aerobes with the "faculty" to switch to anaerobic pathways in the absence of oxygen)	Most human pathogens (e.g., streptococci, entero-bacteria)
Microaerophilic bacteria	Require oxygen but at low levels (**~5% O_2**)	*Campylobacter* *Helicobacter*
Obligate aerobes	Have **only aerobic respiration** and no anaerobic pathways	*Pseudomonas* *M. tuberculosis* *Bacillus*

*The **ABCs** of anaerobiosis are *Actinomyces*, *Bacteroides,* and *Clostridium*. You do not need to know which species are obligate and which are aerotolerant; just learn them as anaerobes.

1. **Viable counts** (colony counts) enumerate only those bacteria that can give rise to a colony. Viable methods give living cell number, not size.

2. **Nonviable methods** (e.g., optical density of the culture, dry cell mass, and quantitative measurement of an individual component) do not distinguish dead cells from living cells.

C. A **growth curve** measures viable bacteria in a broth medium over time. **Figure 3-1B** shows the four stages of a growth curve and the events of each stage. **Figure 3-1C** presents a typical USMLE Step 1 problem. To test yourself, first cover the figure below the heavy line. Remember that there is **only one lag phase,** and that when the cells begin to divide, **one cell always divides into two in each generation.** The answer and explanation for the problem are shown in **Figure 3-1D.**

A.   **Binary Fission**

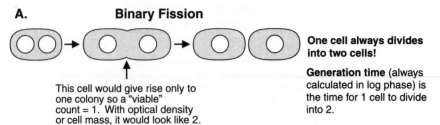

One cell always divides into two cells!

This cell would give rise only to one colony so a "viable" count = 1. With optical density or cell mass, it would look like 2.

Generation time (always calculated in log phase) is the time for 1 cell to divide into 2.

$1 \to 2 \to 4 \to 8 \to 16 \to 32 \to 64 \to 128 \to$ etc

Growth Curve

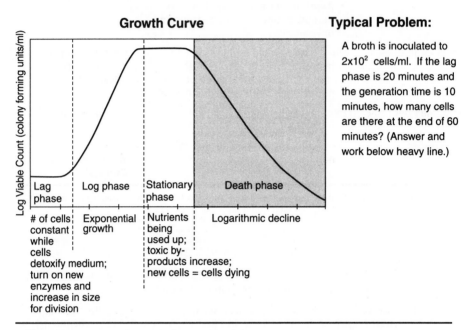

Typical Problem:

A broth is inoculated to 2×10^2 cells/ml. If the lag phase is 20 minutes and the generation time is 10 minutes, how many cells are there at the end of 60 minutes? (Answer and work below heavy line.)

B.   Answer to Growth Curve Problem

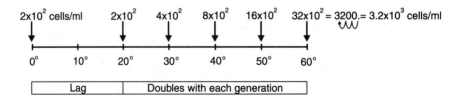

Figure 3-1.   (A) Bacterial growth and division (binary fission, which is asexual). (B) Answer to growth problem in text.

4

Bacterial Pathogenicity

I. INTRODUCTION. Microbial ability to cause disease is complicated and differs for each organism. The resulting disease depends on the natural history of the organism, exposure type and amount, and the microbe's pathogenic mechanisms, as well as the health of the exposed person. Some generalizations are important to review.

II. SURVIVAL IN THE ENVIRONMENT. Most human bacterial pathogens do not survive long in the environment. The more delicate microbes generally are fairly directly transmitted by respiratory droplet spread, direct contact, or living vectors. One or more of the following factors may promote survival of the **hardier pathogens:**

A. Resistance to drying. Spore forms of *Clostridium* and *Bacillus,* the fairly inert environmental forms of *Coxiella* and *Chlamydia,* and the **mycobacteria** with their waxy cell walls all survive drying and may be airborne.

B. Cold growth. Most fecal pathogens die in the cold; however, *Listeria monocytogenes* and *Yersinia enterocolitica* not only survive outside the intestinal tract in the environment, but actually grow at 4°C (39°F).

C. Short-term survival skills. *Staphylococcus aureus* and *Streptococcus pyogenes* are two notable pathogens surviving for short periods of time on fomites. *S. aureus* is spread in hospitals, not only by direct contact, but also on sheets and other fomites.

D. Growth and survival in water

1. *Legionella,* which grows in amebae in streams, contaminates air conditioning cooling tanks and is then spread by air-conditioned air.

2. The opportunist *Pseudomonas* grows well in tap and distilled water and may be found in or on raw vegetables, cut flowers, soil, hot tubs, whirlpools, faucet aerators, and drains.

III. COLONIZATION OF THE HUMAN BODY

A. Colonization by normal flora. Normal flora colonizes the human body's internal and external surfaces. These organisms are **low virulence,** and are generally kept in balance by our surface defense mechanisms.

1. Normal flora **reduces the risk that pathogens will colonize by modifying pH, blocking binding sites,** and **producing** antibacterial compounds called **bacteriocins.**

2. Infection may result if normal flora is carried into normally sterile tissues (e.g., by trauma), particularly in immunocompromised patients.

B. Colonization by pathogens. Some pathogens colonize skin or mucosal surfaces without harm, but may **sometimes invade or cause disease by another mechanism.**

1. **Colonization with further spread to cause disease.** *Streptococcus pneumoniae* colonizes the oropharyngeal mucosa, but is more likely to reach someone's lungs if the cough reflex is suppressed (e.g., in alcoholics) or if the mucociliary elevator is damaged (following influenza or measles). Other pathogens that colonize mucosal surfaces that may cause more invasive disease are *Neisseria gonorrhoeae, N. meningitidis,* and *Haemophilus influenzae* type B.

2. **Colonization with little invasiveness but toxin circulation.** Some bacteria (like *Corynebacterium diphtheriae*) colonize mucosal surfaces and produce toxins, which circulate and cause disease.

3. **Carriers.** A carrier is a colonized or infected individual (generally immune) who harbors a pathogen, but is not ill and who serves as a source to spread the organism to others.

C. Major mechanisms of colonization

1. **Attachment to mucosal surfaces** through bacterial surface molecules
   a. **Gram-positive bacteria** attach to mucosal cell surfaces primarily through the **teichoic acids.**
   b. **Gram-negative bacteria** attach primarily through **pili** and, in some cases, through certain **outer membrane proteins (OMPs).**

2. **Production of an IgA protease.** The Fc fragments produced through the action of these IgA proteases may coat the invading bacterium, allowing it to bind to cells with Fc receptors. The four pathogens listed in the previous section (see **III B 1**) all produce IgA proteases.

3. **Attachment by surface adhesins.** These are mostly proteins (e.g., the M protein of *S. pyogenes* or Gram-negative OMPs).

IV. TRAUMATIC IMPLANTATION INTO THE HUMAN HOST. The intact integument is a major barrier; however, traumatic implantation (e.g., injury, arthropod or animal bites, and sometimes surgery) may allow direct entry of environmental organisms, normal flora organisms (skin or fecal), or pathogens.

V. EVASION OF THE IMMEDIATE HOST DEFENSE SYSTEM

A. **Ability to evade phagocytic uptake** in a nonimmune host is mediated by surface structures. **All bacterial capsules** or slime layers and some pili (notably **N. gonorrhoeae**) are antiphagocytic.

B. **Ability to evade phagocytic killing.** Certain organisms may be phagocytized but not killed. *Listeria* **exits** the phagosome to the cytoplasm quickly enough to avoid damage. Virulent **M. tuberculosis'** sulfolipid (a.k.a. sulfatide) **inhibits** the phagolysosomal **fusion** so M. *tuberculosis* is not killed.

C. **Ability to inhibit ciliastasis or kill ciliated respiratory tract cells.** *Mycoplasma* binds to cilia through P1, an adhesin, causing ciliastasis and, ultimately, desquamation of ciliated respiratory tract cells, which leads to pneumonia.

D. **Ability to resist complement-mediated killing** (a.k.a. membrane activation complex or MAC) occurs with some Gram-negative bacteria and is sometimes referred to as **serum resistance.** MAC resistance may be a result of changes in O antigens of the outer membrane or of sialylation of lipopolysaccharide (LPS).

VI. PRODUCTION OF TOXINS. The **major mechanism** by which extracellular bacteria produce disease is the production of **structural toxins or exotoxins. Details and symptoms** (which you will need for case history questions) are shown in **Table 4-1.**

A. Structural toxins. Endotoxin, produced by Gram-negative bacteria, is the best-studied structural toxin. This is because Gram-negative infections continued to be a problem for several decades despite the introduction of penicillin. Now, because of antibiotic resistance, about half of the cases of septic shock are triggered by Gram-positive bacteria.

    1. Endotoxin. Endotoxin or lipopolysaccharide (**LPS**) is released from the **Gram-negative outer membrane.** Lipid A activates macrophages to produce interleukin-1 (IL-1), IL-6, IL-8, tumor necrosis factor (TNF) alpha, and platelet activating factor. These **cytokines** ultimately stimulate production of prostaglandins and leukotrienes and **activate** both the **complement and coagulation pathways.** Early symptoms are fever, increased number of PMNs in blood, and increased respiratory and heart rates.

    2. Peptidoglycan-teichoic acid. In **Gram-positive cells,** the large fragments of peptidoglycan-teichoic acids from cell walls trigger inflammation and shock through activation of the same chain of events as endotoxin.

B. Exotoxins are generally secreted by living pathogenic bacteria.

    1. Membrane-disrupting bacterial exotoxins
      a. **Pore-forming cytolysins** are protein toxins that are inserted into cholesterol-containing host membranes to create pores. This results in loss of ions and uptake of water, causing the human cell to swell and lyse.
        (1) *Staphylococcus aureus* alpha-toxin and *Streptococcus pyogenes* **streptolysin** are both **pore-forming cytolysins** that destroy a wide variety of cells, including red blood cells.
        (2) **Listeriolysin O** is a **pore-forming toxin** secreted by *Listeria* in the phagosomal environment. It allows *L. monocytogenes* to exit the phagosome into the cytoplasm quickly, so it is undamaged by lysosomal contents.
      b. *Clostridium perfringens* **alpha–toxin,** another cytolysin, is a **lecithinase** that hydrolyzes the eukaryotic membrane phospholipid, destabilizing cytoplasmic membranes. (Alpha-toxin and a second hemolysin called delta-toxin produce *C. perfringens'* characteristic **double zone of hemolysis** on blood agar plates.)

    2. Superantigen exotoxins. Superantigens bind to MHC class II receptors on antigen-presenting cells and cross-link to T-cell receptors, **nonspecifically activating large numbers of T cells.** Excess production of Il-2 and of cytokines leads to shock. The **best known** of the superantigen toxins are **toxic shock syndrome toxin 1 (TSST-1),** produced by some strains of *Staphylococcus aureus,* and the *Streptococcus pyogenes* **exotoxin A (SPE-A).** Both toxins also inhibit normal liver clearance of endotoxin from Gram-negative normal flora, which may play a role in the creation of shock.

    3. A-B (two-) component bacterial exotoxins
      a. ⬤ The **B** component **binds** to specific cell surface receptors and initiates the internalization of the A component. Thus, the B component determines what cell type each toxin damages.
      b. ⬤ The **A** portion of the toxin is the **active toxic portion,** which is **internalized** and then **inhibits** a specific, critical **intracellular function,** thus damaging the cell.
      c. There are **three major classes** of A-B toxins:

Table 4-1

Major Bacterial Toxins: Mechanisms of Action and Effects

	Organism(s)	Toxin(s)	Mechanism of Action	Disease Effect
STRUCTURAL TOXINS—RELEASED ON DEATH OF CELL				
Mediators of inflammation in tissues and of septic shock when in bloodstream	Gram-negative bacteria	Lipopolysaccharides (LPS) = endotoxins. Toxic part is lipid A.	Stimulates host cells to release cytokines IL-1, TNF alpha, IL-6, IL-8, and platelet-activating factors, leading to activation of complement, coagulation, and endothelial damage	Fever, increased respiration and pulse rate, petechial rash leading to ecchymosis, hypotension, thrombocytopenia, internal hemorrhage, and vascular collapse (acute respiratory distress syndrome, disseminated intravascular coagulation, and multiple organ system failure)
	Gram-positive bacteria	Peptidoglycan-teichoic acids. Large pieces of these disintegrating cell wall components trigger the release of the same cytokines as does LPS.	Same as above	Same as above
EXOTOXINS—COMMONLY SECRETED BY LIVING CELLS				
Membrane-disrupting toxins	*Staph. aureus*	Alpha-toxin	Pore-forming cytolysin	Tissue damage, hemolysis
	Strep. pyogenes	Streptolysin O	Pore-forming cytolysin	Tissue damage, hemolysis
	Listeria monocytogenes	Listeriolysin O	Pore-forming cytolysin: rapid egress from phagosome	Survival in human phagocytes, allowing it to spread
	Clostridium perfringens	Alpha-toxin	Lecithinase hydrolyzes eukaryotic phospholipid	Tissue destruction in tissue infections

Category	Organism	Toxin	Mechanism	Effects / Disease
Superantigens, endotoxin enhancers	*Staph. aureus*	Toxic shock syndrome toxin-1 (TSST-1)	TSST-1 enters blood stream, resulting in nonspecific cross-link of major histocompatibility complex and T-cell receptor. This stimulates large numbers of T cells to produce cytokines. Also, there is reduction of liver clearance of endotoxin.	Rash, desquamation of palms and soles, hypotension, capillary leakage, multiorgan failure
	Strep. pyogenes	*Strep. pyogenes* exotoxin-A (SPE-A) [also called erythrogenic toxin, pyrogenic toxin]	Same as for TSST-1; produced only by the most virulent strains	Same as TSST-1 above, with added cardiotoxicity
A–B toxins that inhibit protein synthesis	*Corynebacterium diphtheriae*	Diphtheria toxin	Cells with the most receptors for diphtheria toxin are in the heart and nerves. The A component ADP-ribosylates eukaryotic EF-2 and inhibits protein synthesis.	Sore throat, slight increase in temperature, pseudomembrane in throat, neurologic and cardiac symptoms, death by asphyxiation or heart failure
	Pseudomonas aeruginosa	Exotoxin A	ADP ribosylates EF-2, shutting down protein synthesis primarily in liver cells	Jaundice and increased risk of death in septicemia with exotoxin A-producing strains of *Pseudomonas aeruginosa*
	Shigella dysenteriae type 1	Shiga toxin (ST)	"A" component cleaves 60S ribosomes, inhibiting protein synthesis	Most strains of shigella cause dysentery without producing Shiga toxin. Strains with Shiga toxin do more damage to the colonic mucosa and are more likely to cause hemolytic uremic syndrome (HUS).
	Hemorrhagic *Escherichia coli*	Verotoxin (a Shigalike toxin)	Same as above	Hemorrhagic colitis and HUS
A–B toxins that increase cAMP	Enterotoxic *E. coli* (ETEC)	*E. coli* labile toxin (LT)	Internalized A component ADP-ribosylates G_s, which activates an adenyl cyclase that produces high level of cAMP	Up to 19 L of fluid and electrolytes lost; clear stools with flecks of mucus (rice water stools); major dehydration if not replaced; hypovolemic shock

(continued)

Table 4-1—*Continued*

Major Bacterial Toxins: Mechanisms of Action and Effects

Organism(s)	Toxin(s)	Mechanism of Action	Disease Effect
Bacillus anthracis	Anthrax toxin	Three-component toxin with protective antigen (PA) serving as the B component for either the edema factor (EF) or the lethal factor (LF). The EF is an adenyl cyclase that activates inside cells; the LF kills.	In skin infection, malignant pustules develop with blood fluid vesicles (appearing tumorlike). They become black and necrotic from the center out. In respiratory disease, there is septic shock.
Bordetella pertussis	Pertussis toxin	Pertussis toxin plays a role in the attachment of *B. pertussis* to respiratory mucosa. It also is internalized and inhibits G_i (the negative regulator of adenyl cyclase) through ADP ribosylation. This results in an increase in cAMP.	Increase in respiratory secretions and mucus, decreased phagocytic function in upper respiratory tract, and encephalopathy. The toxin may not be directly responsible for the paroxysmal cough associated with pertussis.
Neurotoxins			
Clostridium tetani	Tetanus toxin	Acts on CNS, inhibiting release of inhibitory transmitters like GABA	Rigid spasm
Clostridium botulinum	Botulinum toxin	Acts on peripheral synapses, blocking release of neurotransmitters	Flaccid paralysis

(1) Inhibitors of protein synthesis
  (a) **Diphtheria** and *Pseudomonas* **exotoxin A toxins** (both EF-2 inhibitors)
  (b) **Shiga toxin** (which cleaves rRNA, inactivating eukaryotic 60S ribosomal subunit) and the nearly identical **Shigalike toxins** (SL-1 and SL-2) and **verotoxin**
(2) Toxins that increase cAMP
  (a) *Escherichia coli* labile toxin (LT)
  (b) Cholera toxin
  (c) Anthrax toxin
  (d) Pertussis toxin
(3) Neurotoxins (both endopeptidases)
  (a) **Tetanospasmin,** producing rigid spasm
  (b) **Botulinum toxin,** producing flaccid paralysis

VII. **INTRACELLULAR GROWTH** gives bacteria some protection from the immune system. Bacteria may kill the host cells by limiting essential components or by interfering with the host cell's respiration.

  A. Bacteria that override killing by macrophages and then **grow inside macrophages** include rickettsias, mycobacteria, *Brucella* spp., and *Listeria*.

  B. Shigellae invade the Peyer's patches through the phagocytic M cells, survive, and exit on the underside. Some shigellae are picked up there and killed by macrophages, but others attach to cellular integrins (only on the basal surface) and invade the columnar mucosal cells. They then can spread laterally by polymerization of actin filaments, which propels them into adjoining cells and creates shallow, lateral ulcers.

5

Bacterial Genetics

I. DNA MOLECULES IN BACTERIAL CELLS. Genes expressed in bacterial cells may be located on one of **three types of DNA molecules:** the bacterial chromosome, plasmid DNA, and stable phage DNA.

   A. Bacterial chromosome (always present). This is most commonly a single **large covalently closed molecule** (~3000 × the diameter of the cell) of typical double-stranded DNA. It is apparently organized into loops and condensed to fit into about 50% of the cell volume. It has **no major histones,** and there is **no nuclear membrane** separating it from the cytoplasm. It contains **all essential bacterial genes.** There may be more than one copy in a cell.

   B. Plasmid DNA. Plasmids are **extrachromosomal pieces of DNA** found sometimes in some bacteria. They are "circular" like bacterial chromosomes, but much smaller.

      1. Functions. Under most growth conditions, plasmid genes are nonessential, but they may be important to **pathogenicity** (through production of bacterial toxins) or to **survival under special conditions** (e.g., in the presence of an antibiotic or chemical).

      2. Types. Fertility factors and **drug resistance factors** are two types of plasmids. Many fertility factors (referred to as **episomes**) can integrate their DNA into the bacterial chromosome. Drug resistance factors generally do not integrate.

   C. Stable phage DNA. A bacterial cell may acquire the third type of DNA, phage (bacterial virus) DNA, through infection with a temperate phage whose viral production is repressed (lysogeny detailed in section III C), or through infection with a defective phage.

II. HOMOLOGOUS RECOMBINATION (STABILIZATION OF NEW GENES). When new bacterial genes enter a bacterial cell by transformation (see III A), they are imported as **linear pieces of DNA (exogenotes).** To avoid rapid degradation by the numerous cellular exonucleases (which attack only free ends of DNA), the new DNA must either circularize (e.g., as plasmid DNA will) or be stabilized into the bacteria's circular chromosome by homologous recombination. **Homologous recombination** (depicted in **Figure 5-1**) is basically **an exchange of two nearly identical pieces of DNA.** The process is complex and **requires a DNA-binding protein called *recA*.** The genes in the covalently closed chromosome survive; the ones on the linear piece are degraded. Homologous recombination is also involved in the stabilization of genes following transduction and conjugation.

Homologous Recombination

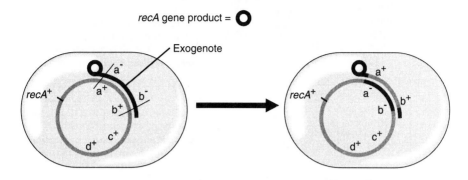

This process is required to stabilize genes introduced by transformation, transduction, and conjugation (except those that circularize). It requires a series of recombination enzymes (represented in all diagrams as the presence of the *recA* gene product).

Figure 5-1. Homologous recombination.

III. GENE TRANSFER (THREE PROCESSES*). Bacterial reproduction is asexual; no new genes are introduced through reproduction, with the exception of an occasional mutation. **Genetic diversity,** an advantage in an ever-changing world (e.g., new antibiotics), is **increased by DNA transfer,** which occurs outside of reproduction. There are three DNA transfer processes: **transformation, conjugation,** and **transduction.**

A. TRANSFORMATION is the binding and uptake of naked extracellular DNA by a competent, living bacterial cell (Figure 5-2). (⬛ Transformation is the <u>transfer</u> of naked <u>forms</u> of DNA.) The recipient cell must be **competent** (i.e., **able to bind the DNA to its surface and bring it in through the cell envelope**) for transformation to occur. Cells become competent under certain environmental conditions (which you do not need to know for USMLE Step 1).

B. CONJUGATION is the transfer of DNA directly from one living bacterium to another. The transfer is **unidirectional** from the "male" donor cell to the "female" recipient. The **cells must physically touch** (they are brought together by sex pili.) This process is under the control of a series of special genes on a **fertility factor** (a plasmid); these genes are called **transfer genes,** or the *tra* operon. Important genes or regions of a typical fertility factor and what they do are shown in **Figure 5-3.** (A quick review of this figure will make the following figures easier to understand.)

    1. Donor cells must have fertility factors. There are two major types of donor cells:
        a. An **F⁺ cell** is defined as a cell with a **free fertility factor** (not inserted into the bacterial chromosome of the cell).
        b. An **Hfr cell** has the **fertility factor inserted** into the bacterial chromosome. It has one large covalently closed molecule of DNA containing both the chromosome and the fertility factor.

---

*The definitions of **transformation, conjugation,** and **transduction** will probably get you through 50% of the bacterial genetic questions. If you want to understand more and score higher, **pay attention to the diagrams.**

Gene Transfer: Bacterial Transformation

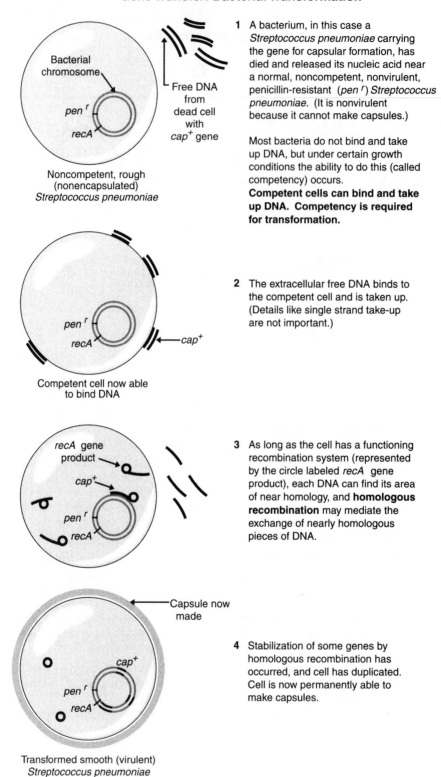

1. A bacterium, in this case a *Streptococcus pneumoniae* carrying the gene for capsular formation, has died and released its nucleic acid near a normal, noncompetent, nonvirulent, penicillin-resistant (*pen*^r) *Streptococcus pneumoniae*. (It is nonvirulent because it cannot make capsules.)

   Most bacteria do not bind and take up DNA, but under certain growth conditions the ability to do this (called competency) occurs. **Competent cells can bind and take up DNA. Competency is required for transformation.**

2. The extracellular free DNA binds to the competent cell and is taken up. (Details like single strand take-up are not important.)

3. As long as the cell has a functioning recombination system (represented by the circle labeled *recA* gene product), each DNA can find its area of near homology, and **homologous recombination** may mediate the exchange of nearly homologous pieces of DNA.

4. Stabilization of some genes by homologous recombination has occurred, and cell has duplicated. Cell is now permanently able to make capsules.

Figure 5-2. Transformation is one of three bacterial DNA transfer processes increasing genetic diversity.

F Factor (a.k.a. F Plasmid or Fertility Factor)
Numbers represent order of conjugal
transfer in approximately 20-second blocks.
Start at *OriT* and study diagram clockwise.

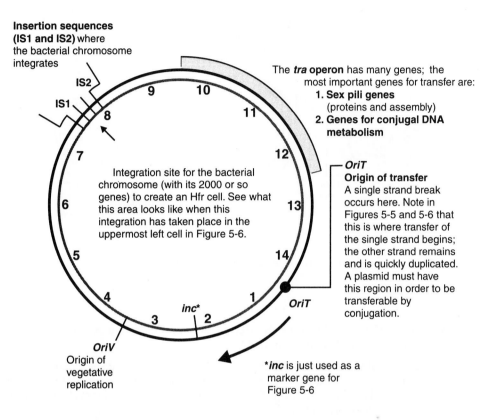

Figure 5-3.   Conjugation: Important genes and regions of a typical fertility factor.

2. **Recipient cells (F⁻ cells) lack fertility factors; they have only the bacterial chromosome.** The recipient in every cross is an F⁻ cell.

3. **Cell types** are diagrammed in **Figure 5-4.**

4. **Two important crosses** are $F^+ \times F^-$ and Hfr $\times$ F⁻.
   a. **$F^+ \times F^-$.** Only a single strand of the plasmid DNA is transferred from the donor to the recipient; the donor genotype stays the same (F⁺), but the **recipient cell** also **becomes F⁺**, as detailed in **Figure 5-5.**
   b. **Hfr $\times$ F⁻.** Because the donor cell fertility factor is integrated into the bacterial chromosome, the fertility factor promotes the single strand transfer of part of the fertility factor and then some of the adjoining bacterial genes (in linear order). **The recipient gets some new bacterial genes but does not become an Hfr cell** (no sex change!) since the whole chromosome is rarely transferred (**Figure 5-6**).

Bacterial Mating Types

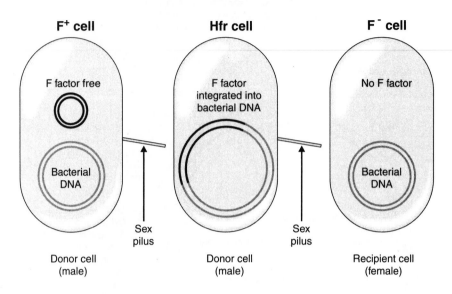

Figure 5-4.   Conjugation: Bacterial mating types.

C. TRANSDUCTION is the transfer of bacterial genes via a bacterial virus (phage) vector (Figures 5-7 through 5-11).

1. **Specialized transducing phage.** If bacterial DNA is picked up when an integrated prophage is being excised, then **only genes adjoining the integration site can be picked up.** Thus, all the phage produced will be specialized transducing phage (**excisional error**) [Figures 5-10 and 5-11].

2. **Generalized transducing phage.** Sometimes during the assembly process, a piece of **bacterial DNA is incorporated into one phage.** Because any gene could be picked up, this is called a generalized transducing phage (**assembly error**). See Figure 5-7, Step 7, and Figure 5-8.

3. **For the USMLE Step 1,** learn the definition of transduction (III C) and study Figures 5-7 through 5-11.

Bacterial Conjugation: F⁺ x F⁻ Mating

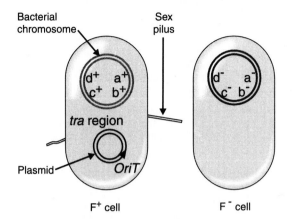

Bacterial chromosome

Sex pilus

d⁺ a⁺
c⁺ b⁺

tra region

Plasmid

OriT

F⁺ cell

d⁻ a⁻
c⁻ b⁻

F⁻ cell

Important points:

1 In the male or F⁺ parent, the fertility factor is present, but free from the bacterial chromosome.

Transfer is unidirectional from male to female.

OriT is transferred first, followed by the rest of the plasmid genes.

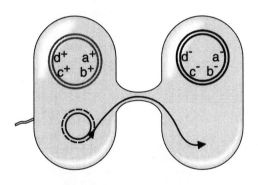

2 Note, only a single strand of the plasmid DNA duplex is transferred.

The area that is lost is reduplicated (shown as dotted lines) so that the donor always stays the same genotype.

The last genes to be transferred are those in the *tra* region.

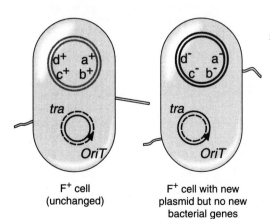

F⁺ cell
(unchanged)

F⁺ cell with new plasmid but no new bacterial genes

3 The transfer of the plasmid is fairly quick, **so assume entire plasmid** is transferred **100%** of the time unless told otherwise.

Note that the F⁻ cell undergoes a sex change, becoming F⁺ (male). These two F⁺ cells can no longer mate.

Note, no BACTERIAL genes are transferred.

Figure 5-5. Conjugation: F⁺ × F⁻ cross.

Bacterial Conjugation: Hfr x F⁻ Cross

Newly synthesized DNA is shown as dashed lines.

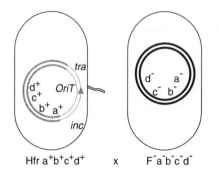

Hfr a⁺b⁺c⁺d⁺   x   F⁻a⁻b⁻c⁻d⁻

<u>Important points:</u>

1 Hfr donor means that the fertility factor (fine line) is already integrated into the bacterial chromosome (heavier grey line).

In this cross, plasmid genes starting at *OriT* will be transferred first, followed by the bacterial genes in linear order away from the plasmid.

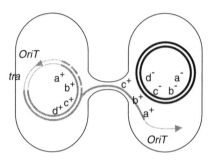

2 Note that as with the F⁺ x F⁻ cross, only a single strand of the DNA duplex is transferred. The area that is transferred is reduplicated (note the rolling model at left) so that the donor always stays the same genotype.

IF the entire chromosome were to be transferred, the last genes to be transferred would be the *tra* region.

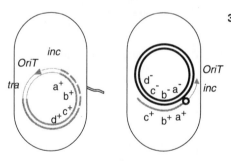

3 It takes approximately 2 hours for a complete transfer to occur. Because the cytoplasmic bridge and DNA are so fine, mating is normally interrupted before the transfer is complete. Assume that mating is interrupted and the recipient gets some new genes but (because it does not get the *tra* operon) does not become Hfr.

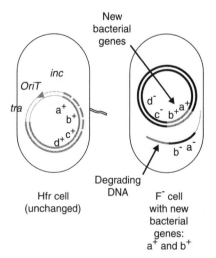

New bacterial genes

Hfr cell (unchanged)

Degrading DNA

F⁻ cell with new bacterial genes: a⁺ and b⁺

Figure 5-6. Conjugation: Hfr × F⁻ cross.

Lytic Replication of Phage

Bacterial virus
= bacteriophage
= phage

=*att*

1 Bacteriophage infects by binding to specific bacterial envelope receptor and injecting DNA. DNA circularizes.

Bacterial DNA
(darker line)

Phage DNA circularizes
(thin line)

Induction of a prophage

2 Early functions: synthesis of mRNAs and proteins to shut off bacterial cell function and to make enzymes and factors to replicate phage DNA.

Early proteins

Early mRNA

3 Phage DNA is synthesized.

4 Late mRNA and proteins (primarily structural proteins) are made.

Phage DNA

5 Assembly

6 Normal infective (non-transducing) phage is released by lysis.

7 This one phage packaged **bacterial DNA** in its head by mistake. It is called a **transducing phage**. Because any gene can be incorporated (depending on what bacterial DNA is incorporated), it is called a **generalized transducing phage.**

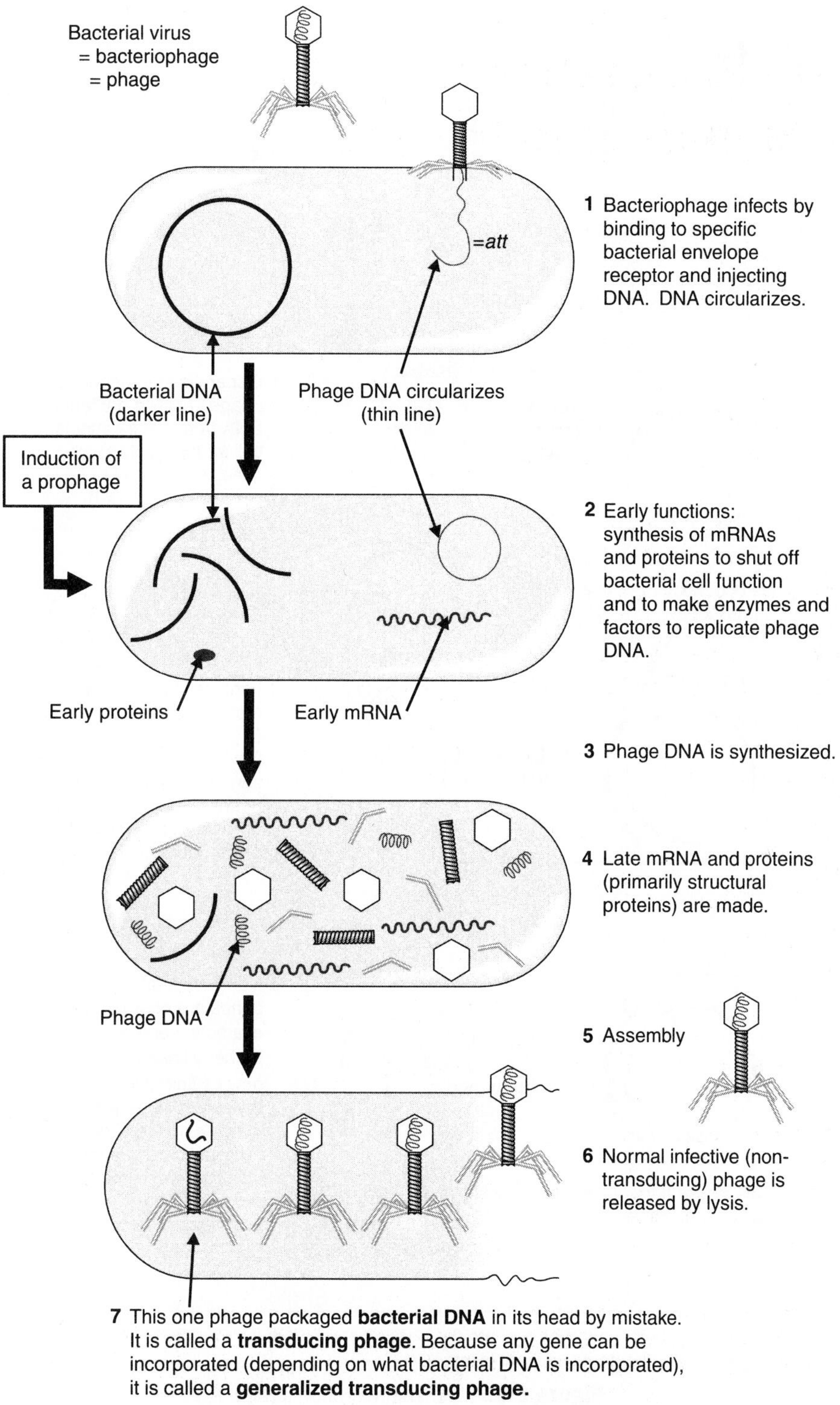

Figure 5-7. Transduction: Lytic replication of phage.

Generalized Transduction

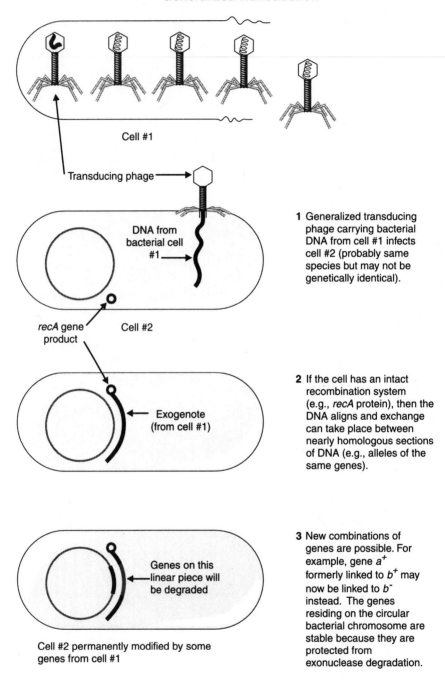

Cell #1

Transducing phage

DNA from bacterial cell #1

recA gene product

Cell #2

1 Generalized transducing phage carrying bacterial DNA from cell #1 infects cell #2 (probably same species but may not be genetically identical).

Exogenote (from cell #1)

2 If the cell has an intact recombination system (e.g., *recA* protein), then the DNA aligns and exchange can take place between nearly homologous sections of DNA (e.g., alleles of the same genes).

Genes on this linear piece will be degraded

3 New combinations of genes are possible. For example, gene a^+ formerly linked to b^+ may now be linked to b^- instead. The genes residing on the circular bacterial chromosome are stable because they are protected from exonuclease degradation.

Cell #2 permanently modified by some genes from cell #1

In generalized transduction, every bacterial gene has an equal chance of being incorporated into the phage head and being transferred to the next bacterial cell that is infected.

Figure 5-8. Generalized transduction.

Temperate Phage and Lysogeny

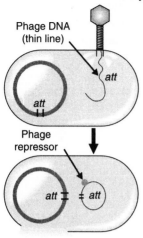

Phage DNA
(thin line)

att

att

Phage
repressor

att ‡ *att*

1 The temperate phage Lambda (λ) is shown. Lambda phage binds to specific receptors and injects DNA, which circularizes.

2 If functional repressor protein is made quickly enough, it inhibits transcription of structural proteins and active production of virus, allowing the virus DNA to integrate.

Phage could have gone into lytic life cycle here if the regulatory battles had gone differently.

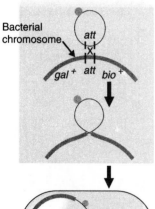

Bacterial
chromosome

att

gal⁺ *att* *bio*⁺

3 Enlarged view of **integration of Lambda DNA**: Note that both molecules of DNA have a small area of homology (*att* sites) where the pairing and crossing over occur. This is a classic example of site-specific recombination where the whole molecule is integrated rather than an exchange taking place. Note that *att* is between the bacterial genes *gal* and *bio*.

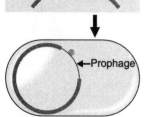

←Prophage

4 This is a **lysogenized cell** (state is called **lysogeny**). When the host bacterial DNA duplicates, so does the phage DNA. As long as the repressor protein continues to be made and is functioning, lysogeny will continue.

5 Prophage integration is somewhat analogous to integration of HIV DNA copy into the human chromosome, where it resides as a provirus.

Figure 5-9. Transduction: Temperate phage and lysogeny.

Induction/excision of prophage leads to:
a. active temperate phage replication or
b. production of specialized transducing phage

If the repressor in a lysogenized cell is damaged by UV light, cold, or alkylating agents, the cell is "induced" into active virus production, which begins with the excision of the prophage DNA. Excision is the reverse of site-specific integration. This is shown below on the left with the normal process and on the right with an occasional error leading to the production of the specialized transducing virus.

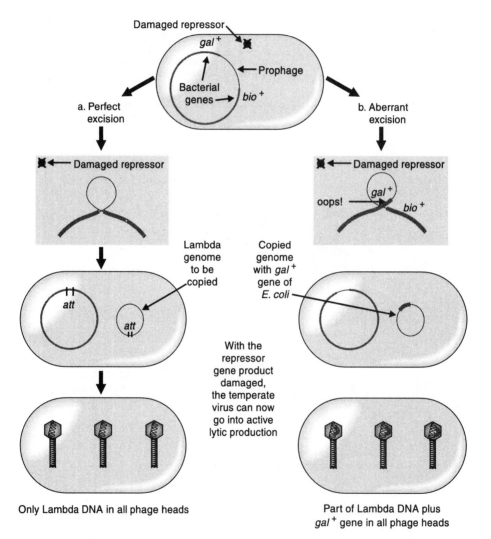

Normal Lambda phage are generally produced. These are not transducing. If after a perfect DNA excision there is a late DNA packaging error, then a generalized transducing phage could be produced along with these normal nontransducing phage.

Specialized Lambda transducing phage are produced, each of which is carrying the *gal*$^+$ gene. (Only the *gal* **or** *bio* genes could have been picked up.)

Figure 5-10. Transduction: Induction/excision of prophage.

Specialized Transduction = Restricted Transduction

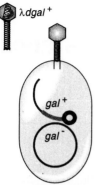

λ*dgal* $^+$

1 Transducing phage created in a *gal* $^+$ cell by induction of a prophage. This defective phage has some Lambda genes and the bacterial gene *gal* $^+$.

gal $^+$

gal $^-$

2 Transducing *gal* $^+$ phage has now injected its DNA into a *gal* $^-$ cell.

E. coli gal $^-$ cell infected with a transducing phage carrying *gal* $^+$

3 If the cell has a functional recombination system, homologous recombination may stabilize some of the genes transferred in. In this case recombination has produced a *gal* $^+$ cell.

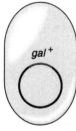

gal $^+$

Summary of Specialized Transduction

1. Specialized transducing phage are produced by an excisional error.

2. Only the genes that adjoin the insertion site (*att*) of a temperate phage can be integrated into the phage.

Now *gal* $^+$

3. Transduced genes must be stabilized by homologous recombination.

Figure 5-11.   Specialized or restricted transduction.

6

Antibiotics and Drug Resistance

I. ANTIBIOTIC MECHANISMS. Antibiotics inhibit cellular processes **or** damage cells. Major antibiotics and their mechanisms are listed in Table 6-1. (See also *High-Yield Pharmacology, Lippincott Williams & Wilkins, 1999.*)

II. ANTIBIOTIC ACTION

A. Bacterio*static* antibiotics **inhibit bacterial growth** while the drug is present.

B. Bacterio*cidal* antibiotics **kill bacterial cells.** Cells do not regrow if the antibiotic is removed.

III. DRUG RESISTANCE MECHANISMS. A variety of alterations in bacterial cell structure or functions lead to drug resistance (DR).

A. Modification of the drug's binding site allows normal cell function to continue even in the presence of the drug. Examples are new penicillin-binding proteins (PBPs) or new ribosome subunits to which the drugs will no longer bind.

B. Reduced access of the drug to binding sites may occur by **decreasing bacterial permeability** (e.g., outer membrane modifications of Gram-negative cells), by **decreasing uptake** of the antibiotic, or by creating an active **efflux pump** (similar to bailing a boat).

C. Antibiotic inactivation occurs through the production of new enzymes, which either **inactivate by adding side groups** (acetyltransferases) or **break critical bonds** (beta-lactamases).

D. For mechanisms of DR, see Table 6-1.

IV. ACQUISITION OF DRUG RESISTANCE

A. Already drug-resistant strains may spread.

1. In nosocomial infections, hospital staff may serve as reservoirs for methicillin-resistant *Staphylococcus aureus* (**MRSA**) or, by improper hygiene, they may transmit MRSA from one patient to the next.

2. Multiple drug-resistant *Neisseria gonorrhoeae* and *Mycobacterium tuberculosis* can spread from contact within the community.

B. DR genes may be transferred from normal flora to a newly acquired pathogen. This is most likely with Enterobacteriaceae in gastrointestinal infections.

C. Resistance and selection may occur through mutation, most notably when a patient is noncompliant during the long antibacterial treatment for tuberculosis.

Table 6-1
Mechanisms of Bacterial Resistance to Antibiotics

	Mechanism of Antibiotic Action	Antibiotics	Mechanisms of Bacterial Resistance
Nucleic acid synthesis inhibition	Inhibition of DNA synthesis DNA gyrase inhibition	Fluoroquinolones	Altered gyrase, reduced permeability
	Electron sink; intermediates damage DNA (anaerobes)	Metronidazole	Uncommon; drug not converted to active form in aerobes
	Folic acid synthesis inhibition	Sulfonamides/trimethoprim	Altered enzymes; reduced permeability or increased efflux
	Inhibition of mRNA synthesis (DNA-dependent RNA polymerase)	Rifampin	Reduced binding to DNA polymerase
Inhibition of protein synthesis and assembly	Action on 50S ribosomal subunit	Macrolides	Methylating enzyme
		Clindamycin	Methylating enzyme
		Chloramphenicol	Acetyltransferase
	Action on 30S ribosomal subunit	Tetracyclines	Increased efflux
		Aminoglycosides	Decreased ribosomal binding; reduced uptake; modifying enzymes
Cell membrane damage	Membrane (outer and cytoplasmic) disrupted	Polymyxins	
Cell wall synthesis inhibition	Early steps in peptidoglycan synthesis	Cycloserine, bacitracin, vancomycin	New, insensitive peptidoglycan precursors
	Cross-linking of peptidoglycan (transpeptidation)	Penicillins/cephalosporins, imipenem, aztreonam	Altered PBP*s; reduced permeability; beta-lactamase

*PBPs = penicillin-binding proteins.

V. GENETICS OF DRUG RESISTANCE

A. **Inherent DR.** Isoniazid inhibits mycolic acid synthesis; however, it inhibits only those few bacteria, like Mycobacteria, that have to make mycolic acid.

B. **Chromosome-mediated DR** commonly involves modification of **the cellular antibiotic–binding site** (e.g., new ribosomes that do not bind antibiotics).

C. **Plasmid-mediated DR. Resistance factors (R factors)** are plasmids with DNA to direct transfer (resistance transfer factor, or RTF) and gene(s) for DR (R-determinant portion).

   1. Plasmids commonly carry genes for new enzymes (e.g., beta-lactamase), which destroy the activity of an antibiotic.

   2. Resistance genes linked to **transposons** are attracted to plasmid insertional "hot spots" (insertion sequences), creating **multiple drug resistance (MDR) plasmids.**

   3. Plasmid genes are easily transmitted by conjugation.

   a. Rapid transfer of **MDR** to another cell is most likely conjugal transfer of MDR plasmid.

   b. **Nonconjugative plasmids** have lost their *tra* region but still **may be transferred by conjugation in a process called "mobilization,"** as long as there is another conjugative plasmid in the cell. (The USMLE loves this paradox!) The most notable example is *N. gonorrhoeae*.

D. There is some transcriptional control of DR genes.

VI. BACTERIA WITH MAJOR DRUG RESISTANCE

A. Gram-positive bacteria

   1. *Enterococcus.* Some strains show vancomycin and streptomycin/gentamicin resistance.

   2. *Staphylococcus aureus.* Some **MRSA** strains are resistant to all drugs in common usage except vancomycin. Methicillin resistance is due to a chromosomal modification of a major PBP; other resistance is due to a MDR plasmid transferred by transduction.

   3. *Streptococcus pneumoniae.* Both low- and high-level penicillin resistance is increasing.

B. Gram-negative bacteria

   1. Enterobacteriaceae. MDR plasmids are transferred by **conjugation.** An example of the promiscuity of bacteria is that MDR plasmids can be transferred from *E. coli* to related pathogens (e.g., *Salmonella*).

   2. N. gonorrhoeae. The beta-lactamase gene resides on nonconjugative plasmids, transferred by conjugation.

   3. *Haemophilus influenzae.* This bacterium has resistance to many antibiotics.

   4. *Pseudomonas.* This organism has inherent resistance (poor porin) and plasmids.

C. Non-Gram-staining bacteria

   1. M. tuberculosis. MDR strains are increasingly common. A patient may acquire an MDR strain or start with a drug-sensitive strain and, through improper adherence to an MDR protocol (i.e., taking too few drugs at a time), may select for DR mutants. Resistance to drugs that bind to ribosomes is particularly common because M. tuberculosis (unlike most bacteria) appears to have only one copy of each of the ribosomal genes.

   2. *Mycoplasma.* This organism has **inherent DR** to all cell-wall active drugs.

7

Identification of Major Bacterial Groups

I. LABORATORY TESTS USED TO IDENTIFY BACTERIA

A. Tests done directly on primary specimens. The tests used depend on the specimen type and may include Gram stain (except where normal flora prevents interpretation), fluorescent antibody staining, dark field microscopy, DNA probe tests, detection of a specific antigen, and specimen culture.

B. Tests done on isolated pure culture. Once grown, the isolated pure culture may be subjected to a variety of tests, including microscopy with differential staining, biochemical assays, and tests to identify specific antigens or nucleic acid sequences.

II. SPECIMENS. Handling specimens properly is critical to successful cultural isolation. Consideration needs to be given to:

A. Collection methods. These are dependent on:

   1. Site of infection. Some sites are more likely to have anaerobes or to have a high risk of contamination with either normal flora or external contaminants.

   2. Most likely organisms to be isolated. For instance, for *Bordetella pertussis*, special calcium alginate or Dacron nasal pharyngeal swabs on wires or cough plates are used.

B. Transport. Some organisms (e.g., staphylococci) are hardy. Others have specific transport needs (e.g., because *Neisseria* is cold intolerant, it is plated on warm chocolate or Thayer-Martin agar as soon as possible).

III. CULTURES

A. Inert broths or agars are used for most bacteria. The choice depends on the specimen site and suspected agent.

   1. Common primary media. Neither is very selective.
      a. Blood agar is a rich agar base supplemented with blood.
      b. Chocolate agar has blood added while the agar is hot enough to lyse the red blood cells.

   2. Specialized selective media promote the growth of specific pathogens (or groups) and inhibit the growth of normal flora.

   3. Differential media allow distinction by appearance between two different colonies of bacteria directly on the plate.

   4. High-yield media (likely to appear in USMLE cases) are listed in **Table 7-1.**

Table 7-1
Selective and Differential Bacterial Culture Media

Medium	Bacteria Isolated and/or Identified
Buffered charcoal-yeast extract (BCYE) agar	*Legionella*
Chocolate agar	*Haemophilus*
	Neisseria from sterile body sites
Eosin-methylene blue agar or MacConkey agar	Enteric bacteria
Hektoen enteric agar	*Salmonella, Shigella* spp.
Loeffler's coagulated serum medium and tellurite medium	*Corynebacterium diphtheriae*
Löwenstein Jensen medium	*Mycobacterium tuberculosis*
Thayer-Martin agar or New York City agar	*Neisseria* from area with normal flora
Regan-Lowe agar medium	*Bordetella pertussis*
TCBS—an alkaline medium	*Vibrio cholerae*

B. **Eukaryotic cell cultures** must be used to culture **chlamydiae,** which are obligate intracellular pathogens and will not grow in cell-free inert media.

C. **No routine culture** is available for **Rickettsiae or *Mycobacterium leprae*** (all obligate intracellular parasites), or for ***Treponema pallidum*** (not intracellular).

D. Incubation atmosphere and temperatures vary depending on the organism to be isolated.

IV. IDENTIFICATION OF BACTERIA

A. **Biochemical tests** detect the presence of specific enzymes, proteins, or cell-wall constituents. Some **enzymes,** which are important because they can be identified with rapid tests or help distinguish major bacterial groups, are shown in **Table 7-2.**

Table 7-2
Important Enzyme Tests Used in Identification of Bacteria

Enzyme	Activity	Bacteria Tested	Test Principle
Oxidase	Cytochrome enzyme	Gram-negative rods— aerobic or facultative anaerobic	Chromogenic test reagent turns black
Catalase	Hydrolyzes hydrogen peroxide to water and oxygen	Differentiates streptococci from staphylococci *Mycobacteria* speciation	Generates O_2 bubbles
Urease	Hydrolyzes urea	Specific bacteria, many involved in UTI	Causes pH change when urea is broken down
Coagulase	Fibrinogen converted to fibrin clot	Speciates staphylococci Identifies *Yersinia pestis*, causative agent of plague	Clots serum

B. Antigens can be identified in specimens or cultures using known antibodies. These tests include enzyme immunoassay (EIA or ELISA) precipitin tests, counterimmuno-electrophoresis (CIE), Western blots, and latex particle agglutination.

C. Stains. Gram stain is an important rapid test. Many other special stains are available to aid in culture identification (e.g., acid fast and fluorescent antibody stains).

D. Gene probes indicate if a particular gene sequence is present (e.g., the gene for vero-toxin production in an *Escherichia coli* strain), but they may require DNA amplification.

V. IMPORTANT BACTERIAL GENERA.

In the past, genus (and species) distinctions were made largely on the basis of biochemical and physical properties of bacteria (e.g., niacin production). Now molecular techniques are also used (e.g., G-C content, ribotyping, and restriction length polymorphisms).

A. Figures 7-1 and 7-2 show characteristics commonly used to distinguish different bacterial genera. These flow charts point out only high-yield differences between organisms that are likely to be used as clues or be tested directly on the USMLE Step 1. Where two or more genera are listed together with no further laboratory indicators, differentiation is generally beyond the scope of the USMLE Step 1.

B. Not all strains of a single bacterial species are identical. For example, O157:H7 strains of *E. coli* (producing verotoxin) may kill a child, even though other strains of *E. coli* are part of the child's normal flora.

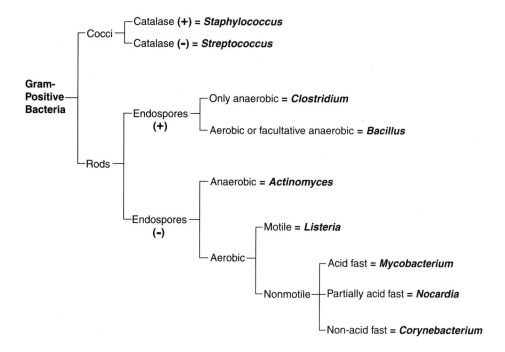

Figure 7-1.   Flow chart for differentiating Gram-positive bacterial genera.

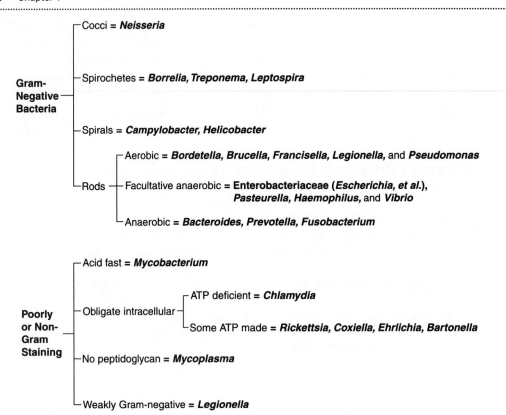

Figure 7-2. Flow chart for differentiating Gram-negative and poorly or non-Gram-staining bacterial genera.

8

Gram-positive Cocci

Staphylococcus, Streptococcus, Enterococcus

I. INTRODUCTION. *Staphylococcus* and *Streptococcus* are the two major genera of disease-causing Gram-positive cocci. **Staphylococci** are **catalase-positive.** Streptococci are **catalase-negative.** (⊕ You can get the word "c a t" from Sta*phyloc̲occus* but not from *Streptococcus.*)

II. STAPHYLOCOCCI. *Staphylococcus* tends to grow in **clusters.** The medically important staphylococci are *S. aureus*, *S. epidermidis*, and *S. saprophyticus*.

A. *Staphylococcus aureus*

   1. Characteristics. *S. aureus* is **coagulase-positive** (initiates formation of fibrin clot), **β-hemolytic,** and **salt-tolerant (haloduric).** *S. aureus* has **protein A** on its surface, which binds Ig Fc (inhibits phagocytosis), produces a yellow pigment, and may produce exotoxins (see A, 5 and 6).

   2. Reservoir and transmission. *S. aureus* resides on human **nasal mucosa** or on the **skin;** it spreads via hands, sneezing, and skin lesions.

   3. Diseases
      a. *S. aureus* **food poisoning** occurs from **heat-stable enterotoxins** produced in poorly refrigerated, *S. aureus*-contaminated foods (e.g., ham, canned or salted meats, custard pastries, or potato salad). Toxin ingestion leads to **rapid onset (1–6 hours) of abdominal pain, vomiting, and diarrhea.**
      b. Skin or subcutaneous infections caused by *S. aureus* present commonly with subcutaneous tenderness and heat, redness, and swelling. Surgery or neutropenia predisposes. Infection may cause exfoliative skin disease (**scalded skin syndrome**) if the strain produces exfoliatins. **Staphylococcal impetigo** generally has **bullae** (large vesicles).
      c. Toxic shock syndrome (TSS). Surgical packing or super tampon use predisposes. **TSST-1,** an exotoxin produced by *S. aureus*, inhibits normal liver clearance of endogenous endotoxin. TSST-1 is also a superantigen activating multiple T helper cells. **Symptoms include fever, hypotension, scarlatiniform rash, desquamation** (particularly on palms and soles), and **multiorgan failure.**
      d. Endocarditis. *S. aureus* **is the dominant cause of acute endocarditis,** including that occurring in IV drug abusers (who often have heavy skin colonization with *S. aureus*.) Alpha toxin (a pore-forming cytolysin) and other cytolytic toxins rapidly damage the heart. Symptoms include fever, malaise, leukocytosis, and development of a heart murmur.

   4. Laboratory identification. *S. aureus* is identified as a Gram-positive staphylococcus that is **beta-hemolytic** and **catalase-** and **coagulase-positive.** The organism grows on **mannitol-salt medium** (the screening medium for *S. aureus*), fermenting the mannitol.

  5. Drug resistance. Methicillin-resistant *S. aureus* (**MRSA**) strains contain a modified major chromosomal penicillin-binding protein (**PBP**). **Most MRSA strains also have plasmid-mediated resistance to all other drugs except glycopeptides (vancomycin).** *S. aureus* drug resistance is transferred by phage (transduction).

B. *Staphylococcus epidermidis*

  1. Characteristics. *S. epidermidis* is **coagulase-negative, nonhemolytic,** and **novobiocin-sensitive** skin flora.

  2. Reservoir. *S. epidermidis* is skin flora.

  3. Diseases. *S. epidermidis* causes **catheter or prosthetic device infections** adhering through production of biofilm. *S. epidermidis* **endocarditis** virtually always occurs in people with indwelling IV catheters or in IV drug abusers; however, *S. aureus* is a far more frequent cause of endocarditis in IV drug abusers.

C. *Staphylococcus saprophyticus*

  1. Characteristics. *S. saprophyticus* is coagulase-negative, nonhemolytic, **novobiocin-resistant,** and normal urethral flora.

  2. Infections. It is one cause of urinary tract infections (**UTIs**) in adolescent (often newly sexually active) females. *S. saprophyticus* UTIs are much **less common than *E. coli* UTIs** in all sexually active women and, unlike *E. coli*, *S. saprophyticus* is nitrite-negative.

III. STREPTOCOCCI. Streptococci are Gram-positive cocci arranged in **pairs or chains;** all are **catalase-negative** and facultative anaerobes. Lancefield's sero*grouping* (Groups A–O) uses known antibodies against cell-wall carbohydrates. Sero*typing* is done on **capsular antigens** (pneumococcus) or **M antigens** (*Strep. pyogenes*). See **Table 8-1.**

A. *Streptococcus pneumoniae*

  1. Characteristics. *Strep. pneumoniae* is a Gram-positive, **lancet-shaped diplococcus.** It is alpha-hemolytic, with growth **inhibited by optochin** and **lysed by bile.**

Table 8-1
High-Yield Streptococci and Enterococci

Species	Lancefield group	Typical Hemolysis	Important Identifiers
Strep. pyogenes	**A**	**Beta**	**Bacitracin–sensitive**
Strep. agalactiae	**B**	**Beta**	**Bacitracin–resistant;** hippurate utilized; incomplete hemolysin (CAMP factor)
Enterococcus faecalis	**D**	Alpha, beta, or none	**Growth in 6.5% NaCl**
Strep. bovis	**D**	Alpha or none	No growth in 6.5% NaCl
Strep. pneumoniae	Not typeable	**Alpha**	**Bile-soluble; Inhibited by optochin**
Viridans group Streptococci	Not typeable	**Alpha**	Not bile-soluble; not inhibited by optochin

2. Virulence factors. Capsule (>80 serotypes, polysaccharide) is antiphagocytic until opsonized. Pneumolysin O (a hemolysin) damages respiratory epithelium. Pneumococcus stimulates outpouring of fluid, RBCs, and leukocytes from alveoli.

3. Reservoir and transmission. Colonization of the nasopharyngeal mucosa (up to 30% of normal people) leads to a respiratory droplet spread; however, *Pneumococcus* is not considered highly contagious because disease rarely occurs in healthy people.

4. Diseases
   a. Pneumococcal pneumonia occurs as a typical **lobar pneumonia** in older adults, alcoholics, and patients with chronic obstructive pulmonary disease (COPD). It is **the major bacterial pneumonia in older adults.**
      (1) Symptoms include rapid onset of chills and fever, and productive cough (blood-tinged or rusty sputum).
      (2) Predisposing factors are **influenza** or other viruses that damage the respiratory mucociliary elevator; **COPD;** and **alcoholism.**
   b. Meningitis. *Strep. pneumoniae* **is the major cause in adults.** Peptidoglycan/teichoic acid elicits a strong inflammatory response in the CNS, resulting in elevated cell counts in CSF.
   c. Otitis media. *Strep. pneumoniae* is the **dominant cause.**

5. Laboratory identification. *Pneumococcus* is an **alpha-hemolytic diplococcus** inhibited by optochin and lysed by bile. It is typed using capsular antibodies. The quellung (capsular swelling) reaction can be used to identify capsule type. Gram stain of CSF sediment and tests for capsular antigen are the rapid diagnostic tests for meningitis.

6. Drug resistance of pneumococci **to penicillins** is increasing.

7. Prevention of infection in people who are asplenic or >65 years old is achieved with the pneumococcal **vaccine.** The vaccine has 23 different capsular serotypes.

B. *Streptococcus pyogenes* **(Group A streptococci or GAS)**

1. Characteristics. *Strep. pyogenes* is a Gram-positive, catalase-negative **coccus occurring in chains;** it is beta-hemolytic and bacitracin-sensitive.

2. Virulence factors include **hyaluronic acid capsule** (antiphagocytic but nonimmunogenic polysaccharide), **M proteins** (surface), **streptolysin O** (immunogenic hemolysin/cytolysin that stimulates anti-streptolysin O or ASO titer), hyaluronidase, C5a peptidase, and kinases that are involved in its ability to spread.

3. Reservoir is the **oropharynx** of **human carriers.**

4. Diseases
   a. "Strep throat." Symptoms are **pharyngitis** with **tonsillar exudate, anterior cervical lymphadenopathy,** fever, and sometimes nausea.
   b. Scarlatina and scarlet fever. "Strep throat" with rash is called scarlatina or, if severe, scarlet fever. *Strep. pyogenes* erythrogenic toxins A-C (**SPE A-C;** a.k.a. pyrogenic toxins) cause fever, rash, T cell proliferation, and B cell suppression. They reduce normal liver clearance of endotoxin from our Gram-negative normal flora. **SPE toxins** are **phage coded.**
   c. Streptococcal impetigo is usually characterized by golden crusted skin lesions (*versus S. aureus* impetigo with bullae).
   d. Necrotizing fasciitis. *Strep. pyogenes'* production of **kinases, hyaluronidase, cytolytic enzymes, SPE A-C, and C5a peptidase** causes a **rapid, life-threatening** infection.

  e. Other *Strep. pyogenes* infections include **erysipelas (infection of dermal lymphatics, usually** of the face), osteomyelitis, and toxic shocklike syndrome.

5. Poststreptococcal sequelae

  a. **Acute glomerulonephritis** (dark urine from hematuria or proteinuria, hypertension, and edema) is **usually an M12 serotype** and a sequela either to pharyngitis *or* to impetigo.

  b. **Rheumatic fever (fever, carditis, subcutaneous nodules, polyarthritis, and chorea)** may follow untreated Group A streptococcal pharyngitis.

6. Laboratory identification

  a. For pharyngitis, **rapid antigen test (if negative, culture);** negative ASO titers on person with repeated positive throat cultures suggest pharyngeal carrier state.

  b. For invasive disease, **culture.**

  c. For rheumatic fever, **ASO titers > 200 are positive.**

7. **Prevention.** Beta-lactams are used as prophylaxis against recurring infections in persons with rheumatic fever who are frequently exposed to children.

C. *Streptococcus agalactiae* (**Group B streptococci, GBS**)

  1. **Characteristics.** *Strep. agalactiae* is a Gram-positive coccus in **chains.** It is beta-hemolytic and bacitracin-resistant. The major **virulence factor** is **polysaccharide capsule.**

  2. **Reservoir.** *Strep. agalactiae* colonizes GU and GI tracts.

  3. Infections

   a. **In adults,** GBS can cause symptomatic fever; it can also cause UTI in pregnant women, leading to amnionitis or endometritis.

   b. **In neonates,** GBS has two presentations: **early onset** (1–7 days), characterized by respiratory problems, sepsis, pneumonia, and meningitis; and **late onset,** characterized by septicemia and meningitis. Penicillin administered to pregnant women with fever of unknown origin, GBS UTI, delivery at <37 weeks, or membrane rupture ≥ 18 hours can reduce the incidence of neonatal disease.

D. Viridans streptococci (*Strep. salivarius, Strep. mutans, Strep. sanguis,* etc.)

  1. **Characteristics.** These streptococci are alpha-hemolytic (partial/"green") and insensitive to bile and optochin. They are **normal** oral, GI, and GU tract **flora.**

  2. **Diseases.** Endocarditis (generally subacute) may follow dental trauma in persons with previously damaged valves. *Strep. mutans* **causes dental plaque and decay through production of dextran biofilm and acids that damage dental enamel.**

IV. **ENTEROCOCCI.** *Enterococcus faecalis* and *Enterococcus faecium* are found in the **GI tract** and **vagina.** They cause **UTIs** and **subacute endocarditis** in patients with previously damaged hearts following urinary or GI tract manipulations. Some strains are **resistant to vancomycin.**

9

Gram-Positive Bacilli

Bacillus, Clostridium, Listeria, Corynebacterium, Actinomyces, Nocardia, Mycobacterium

I. **MAJOR GENERA.** Major genera of Gram-positive bacilli are listed with some of their distinguishing characteristics in **Table 9-1.**

II. ***BACILLUS.*** This genus consists of **Gram-positive,** aerobic **spore formers.**

    A. *Bacillus anthracis*

        1. Transmission. Spores remain in the environment (soil, animal skins) and may be traumatically implanted or inhaled.

        2. Virulence factors
            a. Polypeptide (poly-D-glutamate) capsule (immunogenic and antiphagocytic)
            b. Anthrax toxin, a three-component exotoxin:
                (1) Protective antigen (equivalent to a B component) binds to cells and facilitates the entry of either lethal factor or edema factor.
                (2) Lethal factor kills cells by an unknown mode of action.
                (3) Edema factor is a calmodulin-activated adenylate cyclase.

        3. Infections
            a. Cutaneous anthrax (hazard for people working with hooved animals, their skins, or wool). Traumatic implantation of spores leads to a raised red tumor-like lesion, which progresses to a black, necrotic lesion (eschar) with a red, rolled edge. Systemic symptoms are minimal.
            b. Anthrax pneumonia (wool sorter's disease) is a rapid, life-threatening pneumonia if not treated promptly.

    B. *Bacillus cereus* occurs naturally in rice and vegetables. The spores are not killed by boiling; when rice is made into a higher protein food (typically fried rice) and poorly held and refrigerated, toxins are produced. When reheated and ingested, the toxins cause rapid (1–6 hours) nausea, vomiting, and diarrhea similar to symptoms from staphylococcal food poisoning.

III. ***CLOSTRIDIUM.*** This genus consists of large, Gram-positive, **anaerobic spore–forming rods.**

    A. *Clostridium tetani*

        1. Reservoir and transmission. C. *tetani* is a soil spore former. Traumatic implantation into tissues with low oxygenation (e.g., via puncture wounds, burn wounds,

Table 9-1
Differentiation of Gram-positive Bacilli and Branching Bacteria

Genus	Spores?	Oxygen Utilization*	Acid-fast?	Other Features
Bacillus	Yes	Aerobe	No	
Clostridium	Yes	Anaerobe	No	
Listeria	No	Aerobe	No	Intracellular; tumbling motility
Corynebacterium	No	Aerobe	No	
Actinomyces	No	Anaerobe	No	
Nocardia	No	Aerobe	Partial; yes	
Mycobacterium	No	Aerobe	Yes	Poorly Gram staining Often intracellular in tissue

*Note: There are species variations with respect to growth conditions. For the USMLE Step 1, work with the large picture only.

unsterile surgery, or deliveries) leads to spore germination, growth, and toxin production.

2. Infection/toxicity. Tetanus toxin, a neurotoxic exotoxin, acts on anterior horn cells, blocking release of inhibitory mediators (glycine and GABA) and resulting in rigid spasm. Spastic paralysis begins in the jaw area (**trismus,** lockjaw, **risus sardonicus**) and descends, if untreated, causing paralysis of large muscle groups including **opisthotonos** (rigid back spasm) and death from **paralysis of throat and respiratory muscles.**
  a. **Treatment** of symptomatic tetanus includes:
    (1) **Tetanus immune globulin (TIG)** at the wound site
    (2) **Vaccination** with either the active tetanus-diphtheria vaccine (> 7 years of age); or diphtheria-tetanus-pertussis (DTaP or DTP) (< 7 years of age).
    (3) **Spasmolytic drugs**
    (4) **Metronidazole or penicillin**
  b. **Prevention**
    (1) The tetanus **vaccine** (**toxoid,** the inactivated toxin) is given at 2, 4, 6, and 18 months; at 5 years; and then as a booster every 10 years.
    (2) **Wound prophylaxis** involves proper wound care plus the treatment listed in **Table 9-2.**

Table 9-2
Prophylactic Treatment Against Tetanus

Patient's Vaccination Status	Minor, New Wounds with Healthy Surrounding Tissue	More Serious Wounds
Unknown or not completed primary series of three	Vaccine	TIG* around site *and* vaccine
Completed primary vaccination series	No vaccine unless >10 years since last vaccination, then give booster	Booster if >5 years since last inoculation

*TIG is human tetanus immunoglobin.

B. *Clostridium perfringens*

1. Reservoir and transmission. *Cl. perfringens* is a large spore former found in **soil, dust,** and **feces.** It causes wound infections and food poisoning (via reheated meat dishes).

2. Myonecrosis (gas gangrene) is mixed anaerobic cellulitis in tissues with compromised oxygen supply. *Cl. perfringens'* numerous toxins cause **pain, massive tissue destruction with production of gas, and shock.** Tissue destruction is largely a result of **alpha toxin** (a.k.a. phospholipase C), a lecithinase that destroys eukaryotic membranes. Theta toxin destroys PMNs. Fermentation of muscle carbohydrates produces gases. The infection is rapidly fatal if not treated.

    a. Diagnosis is made by visualizing Gram-positive bacilli in tissues with sparse PMNs; infection is confirmed by anaerobic cultures.

    b. Treatment is by debridement, use of hyperbaric chamber, management of shock, plus penicillin and clindamycin.

3. *Cl. perfringens* **food poisoning** presents with **secretory diarrhea** with acute mid-epigastric **cramping** 8 to 24 hours after ingestion of heavily contaminated meats (usually prepared in large quantities and kept warm, not hot, for an extended time). It resolves within 24 hours.

C. *Clostridium botulinum.* This **neurotoxic** spore former, found in **soil and dust,** causes botulism.

1. Food-borne botulism (toxicosis)

    a. Reservoir and transmission. The toxin is produced in poorly canned **alkaline vegetables** (e.g., green beans, mushrooms). If the contaminated food is not heated thoroughly to 60°C (140°F) to inactivate the toxin (or not heated at all as in **five-bean salad), the botulinum toxin is absorbed in the gut** and acts on the myoneuronal junctions, **blocking release of acetylcholine.**

    b. Clinical manifestations. Incubation is one to two days, followed by early symptoms like **double vision, diplopia,** and **dry mouth,** and then by **symmetric, descending paralysis.**

    c. Diagnosis is made by demonstration of toxin in remaining food, serum, or stool and by culture of stool or food.

    d. Treatment. Patients require supportive care, plus **hyperimmune human globulin.**

2. Infant botulism (a toxi-infection)

    a. Reservoir and transmission. Infants ingest spores (found in **dust or honey**). The immature GI tract flora permits germination of the *Cl. botulinum* spores; **toxin is produced in the GI tract.**

    b. Symptoms include **constipation** and **generalized weakness,** with weak crying, poor feeding, lethargy, and loss of head control **(floppy baby syndrome),** and can lead to **respiratory arrest.**

    c. Treatment. Monitoring with supportive care leads to complete recovery. **Hyperimmune human immunoglobulin** is used. **Antibiotics are generally not used;** they may prolong the infection by preventing development of normal flora.

3. Wound botulism (toxi-infection of a sterile site) is infection of tissue with production of botulinum toxin; treat with **antibiotics and hyperimmune serum.**

D. *Clostridium difficile*

1. Reservoir. This **anaerobic spore former** is found in **soil and** the **human GI tract.** *Cl. difficile* overgrowth of the GI tract is often associated with **antibiotic use.**

2. **Toxins** are polypeptides A (an enterotoxin) and B (a cytotoxin causing cytoskeleton changes in tissue culture cells).

3. **Symptoms of infection** range from **mild diarrhea to pseudomembranous colitis** (abdominal cramping, fever, and diarrhea containing blood and pus).

4. **Treatment** is with **metronidazole** (*not* vancomycin, to avoid vancomycin resistance).

IV. *LISTERIA.* This genus consists of Gram-positive rods with **tumbling motility** and **cold growth** (rare in pathogens). *Listeria monocytogenes,* the important pathogenic species in humans, is a **facultative intracellular** species. It grows in nonimmune macrophages and cells lining the GI tract.

   A. **Reservoir and transmission.** *L. monocytogenes* is found in the **GI tract of animals** and survives in soil. It is **food-borne** in cabbage, deli meats, and some soft cheeses.

   B. **Virulence factors.** *L. monocytogenes* is **invasive;** listeriolysin permits *Listeria* to escape the phagosome before lysosome-phagosome fusion occurs. *Listeria* moves laterally cell to cell by polymerization of actin filaments, propelling the *Listeria* into the adjoining cell.

   C. Infections

      1. **Mild gastroenteritis,** generally in the summer. Some people remain fecal carriers.

      2. **Septicemia in pregnant women.** *Listeria* can cross the placenta to cause **granulomatosis infantiseptica;** it can also contaminate the birth canal and cause neonatal septicemia or, rarely, **neonatal meningitis.**

      3. **Meningitis in immunocompromised patients,** particularly **renal transplant patients,** is the most common clinical listeriosis.

V. *CORYNEBACTERIUM.* This genus consists of Gram-positive, **club-shaped,** nonmotile **rods** that grow best in oxygen. **C.** *diphtheriae* is the major pathogen.

   A. **Reservoir and transmission.** *C. diphtheriae* has **human reservoirs,** with **respiratory spread.** It colonizes but does not invade the oropharynx.

   B. **Virulence** is due to **diphtheria toxin** production and toxin circulation. Diphtheria toxin (an A-B toxin) is an ADP ribosyl transferase that binds to eukaryotic elongation factor-2 (EF-2), **inhibiting protein synthesis.** Diphtheria toxin's B (binding) component "directs" the toxin primarily to the oropharyngeal mucosa, **heart, and nerve cells.**

   C. **Symptoms of infection. Diphtheria symptoms** are **pharyngitis** with **dirty white pseudomembrane** (dead cells, fibrin, and grey pigment), "bull neck" (**cervical lymphadenitis**), **myocarditis, cardiac dysfunction, and laryngeal nerve palsy.** Death may occur from respiratory obstruction or cardiac failure.

   D. **Prevention** of infection is accomplished by vaccination with **diphtheria toxoid.**

   E. Treatment requires both **antitoxin** *and* **antibiotic** (erythromycin or penicillin).

VI. *ACTINOMYCES.* This genus consists of Gram-positive, **non-acid-fast, anaerobic** bacteria that vary **from rods to branching filamentous forms.**

   A. **Reservoir.** *Actinomyces* are **normal bacterial mucosal flora** found in **gingival crevices** and the **female genital tract.**

   B. **Infections.** Endogenous infections arise from trauma to tissues that compromises blood flow to tissues and allows *Actinomyces* to penetrate. A. *israeli* (the major pathogen) grows without respect for internal anatomic barriers. Disease is usually **cervicofacial** ("lumpy jaw" from tooth extraction), thoracic, or abdominal (e.g., from intrauterine devices). Symptoms include **abscesses, swelling,** and, ultimately, **sinus tract formation** with hard, yellowish **microcolonies called "sulfur granules."** Brain abscesses can also occur.

C. **Treatment** with an **antibacterial agent** (usually penicillin) is generally slow but successful.

VII. *NOCARDIA.* This genus consists of **Gram-positive, aerobic, partially acid-fast filaments** that break up into rods. These are hardy organisms found in soil.

A. **Pulmonary nocardiosis** (acquired by inhalation) occurs in patients with low WBC or CD4+ counts. Infections resemble tuberculosis with hematogenous spread to other organs, including the brain.

B. **Cutaneous or subcutaneous infections** may be caused by traumatic implantation.

C. **Brain abscesses** can be caused by both *Nocardia* and *Actinomyces*. (See **Table 9-1** to distinguish these two organisms.)

VIII. *MYCOBACTERIUM.* This genus consists of poorly Gram staining, obligate aerobic bacilli. Mycobacteria are **acid-fast** (because of the very waxy and hydrophobic arabinogalactan-mycolate cell wall layer), and are generally **intracellular.**

A. *Mycobacterium tuberculosis* **(M. tb.)** is a facultative intracellular, human pathogen that causes tuberculosis (TB). M. *tb.* is a major problem among the poor and HIV positive in crowded urban living situations, because of increased chance of respiratory spread and presence of untreated patients.

1. **Virulence** is dependent on two compounds in the waxy M. *tb.* cell envelope. **Cord factor (trehalose mycolate)** inhibits mitochondrial respiration (and, in culture, causes virulent M. *tb.* to grow as serpentine cords). **Sulfolipids** (a.k.a. sulfatides) **inhibit phagosome-lysosome fusion,** allowing M. *tuberculosis* to survive intracellularly.

2. **Culture.** Standard media used to culture M. *tb.* include **Lowenstein-Jensen,** Middlebrook, and broths for rapid automated systems. **M. *tb.* produces niacin** (most other mycobacteria do not). It has a heat-sensitive catalase, so **in the standard catalase test** run at 68°C (154°F), **it is catalase-negative.** Antibiotic susceptibility testing is important.

3. **Exposure, infection, and disease (TB).** Typically, a healthy person who is infected with M. *tb.* has limited replication of the organism in a lung "spot" and adjoining lymph node, both of which are "healed" off in **granulomas** (the Ghon complex) without active disease symptoms. The organism's growth is slowed down by the reduced oxygen level, but M. *tb.* remains viable without prophylactic isoniazid. Without prophylaxis, if one of the granulomas erodes later in life (freeing the organisms into higher levels of oxygen) *and* the person's immune system is suppressed, reactivational (secondary) TB occurs. If initially a person's immune system is unable to contain the infection, contiguous spread (sometimes with cavitary disease) may result. **Hematogenous dissemination** results in systemic disease **(miliary TB).**

4. **Diagnostic tools**
   a. **Purified protein derivative (PPD) skin test.** In tuberculin skin testing with 5TU PPD, **induration** is read at 48 to 72 hours. A level of ≥10 mm or more is positive in a person with risk of exposure; ≥5 mm is positive in HIV-posi-

tive patients; however, **a positive PPD test only indicates exposure;** it cannot, by itself, distinguish exposure from active disease and, in patients with overwhelming disease, the test may be negative.

   b. **Chest auscultation and x-ray,** along with clinical symptoms, aid diagnosis.

   c. **Sputum microscopy.** Rhodamine-auramine stain of clinical specimens (e.g., sputum) is used; this is a sensitive fluorescent dye that binds to the waxy cell wall of the mycobacteria, but it is not specific because no antibodies are involved. If rhodamine-auramine stain is positive, confirm with acid-fast stain; culture the sputum for mycobacteria and run drug susceptibilities.

5. **Treatment for active TB** always involves use of **multiple drugs.** (M. *tb.* develops drug resistance rapidly when treated with a single drug.)

   a. **Uncomplicated pulmonary tuberculosis.** Current standard protocol is to **start with three drugs** (isoniazid [INH], rifampin [RIF], and pyrazinamide) for two months, and then to cut back to INH and RIF for four more months or until sputum smear and culture are negative for two consecutive months.

   b. **Reasonable risk of infection with multiple-drug-resistant TB.** Ethambutol or streptomycin is added to the above regimen for the first two months.

6. **Prophylaxis for recent tuberculin skin test converters** under 35 years of age is **isoniazid** for six to nine months.

B. *Mycobacterium avium-intracellulare.* This **soil or water** organism is an **opportunist** that causes infection in compromised hosts. **Pulmonary infections** occur in patients with cancer, organ transplant, and AIDS, and are similar to TB. M. *avium-intracellulare* is **not contagious from person to person. Prophylaxis** is routine in AIDS patients when CD4+ cells are ≥50/cu mm.

C. *Mycobacterium marinum* is a marine aerobe causing **fish tank granulomas.**

D. *Mycobacterium leprae.* This **obligate intracellular parasite** (no culture), invades skin, peripheral nerves, and, in lepromatous leprosy, upper airways and nasal mucosa. **Humans** are the **only significant reservoir** (there are some infected armadillos). **Leprosy** is a disease with a spectrum of symptoms. Features of the two extreme forms are presented in **Table 9-3.**

Table 9-3
Tuberculoid vs Lepromatous Leprosy

Distinguishing Features	Tuberculoid Leprosy	Lepromatous Leprosy
Cell-mediated immunity	Strong CMI	Weak CMI
Lepromin skin test	Lepromin-positive	Lepromin-negative
Tissue *M. leprae* (as seen in acid-fast stained punch biopsy)	Few acid-fast bacilli (AFB) seen	Many AFB seen (foam cells filled) More contagious
Symptoms	• One to few flat lesions • Nerve enlargement • Loss of sensation leads to burns, trauma	• More severe disease • Multiple, bilaterally distributed skin lesions (often nodular) • Leonine facies

10

Non-Gram Staining or Poorly Gram Staining Bacteria

Non-Gram Staining: *Mycoplasma, Ureaplasma*
Poorly Staining: *Mycobacterium,* Spirochetes, *Rickettsia, Chlamydia, Legionella*

I. NON-GRAM STAINING BACTERIA

A. *Mycoplasma.* Mycoplasmata are bacteria that permanently lack **peptidoglycan.** Mycoplasmata incorporate **sterols** into their membranes but cannot make them, so they are cultured on special media (Mycoplasma, Eaton's). They are the **smallest free-living bacteria,** and are not seen on Gram stain.

  1. *Mycoplasma pneumoniae* is an extracellular human pathogen with **respiratory spread.** It attaches via P1 protein to the respiratory epithelium and secretes hydrogen peroxide, superoxide radical, and cytolytic enzymes, leading to necrosis of the respiratory epithelium.

   a. Infections. M. *pneumoniae* causes sore throat, bronchitis, or otitis media (all without coryza). It spreads down the respiratory tract to cause **atypical pneumonia** (often referred to as "walking pneumonia") characterized by **fever, malaise ± headache,** and **hacking cough** (initially dry, later productive), which lasts up to 4 weeks. **Mycoplasmas** are the **leading cause of pneumonia in school-aged children and young adults,** but can infect individuals of any age. (Viral pneumonia predominates in infants, and *Streptococcus pneumoniae* in adults over 65 years of age.)

   b. Diagnosis is still largely **clinical** since culture is slow and available tests are insensitive. Complement fixation titers ≥1:32 strongly suggest infection. About 65% of the patients produce **cryoagglutinins** (which agglutinate RBCs in the cold); this is suggestive but not specific.

   c. Treatment is with macrolide or tetracycline, **not beta-lactam antibiotics.**

  2. *Mycoplasma hominis* is a genito-uropathogen.

B. *Ureaplasma urealyticum.* This bacterium is also missing a cell wall. It **metabolizes urea,** and causes urethritis and prostatitis.

II. POORLY GRAM STAINING OR POORLY VISIBLE BACTERIA. Gram dyes penetrate the cell peptidoglycan and get trapped inside.

A. **Mycobacteria** don't take up the stain well because of their waxy cell wall, but they are basically Gram-positive (no outer membrane or LPS).

B. Several Gram-negative organisms are so thin that the stain color cannot be seen, but they do have a Gram-negative envelope (e.g., **spirochetes, rickettsias, and chlamydiae**). *Legionella* stains Gram-negative only if the counterstain time is increased.

11

Gram-Negative Cocci

Neisseria, Moraxella

I. *NEISSERIA.* This genus consists of **Gram-negative, kidney-bean-shaped diplococci** that are **oxidase-positive.** The **oxidase test** is important because it is simple and fast and, if positive, it **rules out** that the Gram-negative organism is an **Enterobacteriaceae.** The reagent (phenylenediamine) **quickly turns black** if the tested colony is producing cytochrome C oxidase.

A. *Neisseria meningitidis* (Figure 11-1)

   1. Virulence factors. The capsule is the major virulence factor; it reduces splenic clearance of *N. meningitidis* from the blood by reducing phagocytic uptake and complement activation. *N. meningitidis* B and C are the most common serotypes in the U.S. *N. meningitidis* produces **excess outer membrane fragments** (more than can be incorporated), which is why it is such a **potent inducer of skin rash, inflammation, and shock.**

   2. Reservoir and transmission. The only reservoir is the **human nasopharynx;** transmission is by **respiratory spread.** To get into the meninges, bacteria that have colonized the mucosa must then invade into the blood stream.

   3. Infection. Meningococcemia is characterized by acute onset of fever and rash, rapid decline to coma, and Gram-negative shock.

   4. Laboratory identification. Gram stain or capsular antigens tests (usually a latex particle agglutination) may rapidly detect *N. meningitidis.* CSF sediment is plated on chocolate agar; **N. *meningitidis* ferments maltose.** (*Note:* Nasopharyngeal cultures of close contacts in an outbreak are plated on Thayer-Martin; nonpathogenic strains of *Neisseria,* which are found in the upper respiratory and GU tracts, do not grow on Thayer-Martin medium.)

   5. Prevention of infection
   a. Vaccination against *N. meningitidis* is routine in the military. In outbreaks in the general population, close contacts are vaccinated. The vaccine has four serotypes of capsule: Y, W-135, C, and A (● **YWCA vaccine).** B capsule (which is sialic acid) is not strongly immunogenic.
   b. Rifampin, which reduces mucosal colonization, is also used to reduce risk of disease in close contacts.

B. *Neisseria gonorrhoeae*

   1. Characteristics. *N. gonorrhoeae* is a Gram-negative diplococcus with flattened sides; it is oxidase-positive and has **no capsule.**

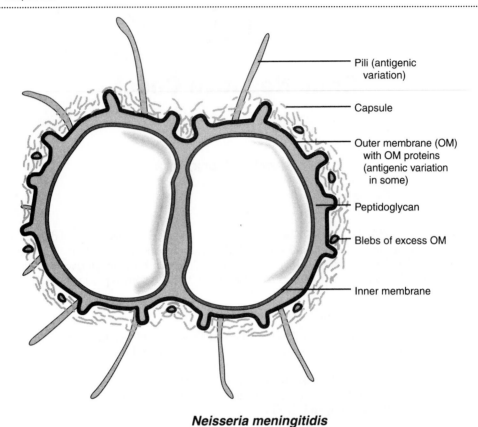

Neisseria meningitidis

Figure 11-1. *Neisseria meningitidis* has both capsule and excess outer membrane fragments.

2. **Virulence factors**
   a. **Pili** play a major role in attachment to mucosal surfaces. Pili have constant and hypervariable regions (**>1 million piliated variants**); hence, there is no immunity to reinfection.
   b. **IgA protease** aids in colonization.
   c. **Outer membrane proteins. Protein I** (a porin protein) is associated with virulence. **Opa (opacity) proteins** increase adherence of bacteria to each other.
   d. **Endotoxin.** *N. gonorrhoeae* invades mucosal surfaces and causes inflammation.

3. **Reservoir and transmission.** *N. gonorrhoeae* colonizes human mucosa, most commonly the genital tract. Transmission is via sexual contact or passage through an infected birth canal.

4. **Infections. Gonorrhea.** (Note: There are frequent coinfections with chlamydiae.)
   a. **Males** present with **urethritis** or **epididymitis.** Male homosexuals (or anyone practicing oral or anal sex) may present with **anorectal lesions** or **pharyngitis.**
   b. **Females** may have **endocervicitis** or **PID,** which often goes undiagnosed. If *N. gonorrhoeae* is not treated, it may disseminate hematogenously, causing **arthritis** in large weightbearing joints and **rash.**

   c. **Infants** present with **hyperpurulent ophthalmia,** which leads to rapid loss of eyesight if not treated.

5. **Laboratory identification.** Tests include nucleic acid **probes and polymerase chain reaction,** microscopy looking for intracellular Gram-negative organisms in neutrophils (useful with male urethral exudate), and **cultures on Thayer-Martin** (in candle jar or Gas Pak for high CO_2).

6. **Drug resistance.** Plasmid-encoded penicillinase TEM-1 causing high-level resistance has been found, primarily in some Southeast Asian strains.

7. **Prevention.** In neonates, silver nitrate or erythromycin in the eyes is used to prevent infection.

8. **Treatment. Ceftriaxone** is used for treatment; azithromycin or doxycycline is added if coinfection with *Chlamydia trachomatis* is not ruled out.

II. *MORAXELLA*

A. **Characteristics.** *Moraxella* is a genus of Gram-negative diplococci found in the upper respiratory tract as normal flora. The most significant human pathogen is *Moraxella catarrhalis*.

B. **Infections.** *M. catarrhalis* is seen in **otitis media** and may cause **bronchitis** in patients with COPD.

12

Gram-Negative Aerobic Bacilli

Pseudomonas, Legionella, Bordetella, Francisella, Brucella

I. *PSEUDOMONAS*

A. Characteristics. This genus consists of **Gram-negative, catalase-positive rods** that are motile and ubiquitous (common in water and soil). *Pseudomonas aeruginosa* (an important opportunist) is medically most important. *Ps. aeruginosa* has a distinctive **grape-like odor** and produces pigments: **pyocyanin,** responsible for **blue-green pus** in burn patients' wounds, and **fluorescein.**

B. Virulence factors. *Pseudomonas* has a slime layer (**capsule**), **exotoxin A** (an ADP-ribosyl transferase that inactivates EF-2, shutting down protein synthesis primarily in liver cells), catalase, pigments, endotoxin, and an **elastase,** which damages immunoglobulins, elastin, and some collagens.

C. Reservoirs. Hospital sources are such things as water faucet aerators, drains, respiratory equipment, raw vegetables, flowers, slimy bar soap, and standing water (distilled or tap).

D. Infections in susceptible patients. Exposure to *Pseudomonas* is so common that at any point in time about 10% of the normal population has transient *Pseudomonas* GI tract colonization (resulting only in loose stools). This incidence rises as high as 70% in hospitalized patients on antibiotics.

1. Normal noncompromised people: hot tub folliculitis (inflamed hair follicles from the neck down); **eye ulcers** from trauma or extended wear of contact lenses; **foot wounds** (e.g., puncture wounds **through soles of tennis shoes,** a *Ps. aeruginosa* haven!); **swimmer's ear**

2. Burn patients: cellulitis and septicemia. GI tract colonization, often from raw vegetables or poor disinfection of equipment like respirators or whirlpools, leads to colonization of burns and may result in frank cellulitis with **blue-green pus** and septicemia. Symptoms of *Ps. aeruginosa* septicemia include fever $+/-$ target lesions (**ecthyma gangrenosum:** black necrotic center with a raised erythematous margin), and may progress to Gram-negative shock and death.

3. Cystic fibrosis (CF) patients: pulmonary colonization with *Ps. aeruginosa* occurs early in CF patients and is difficult to eradicate, because microcolonies are protected in the capsular slime. **Repeated pneumonias** are common, and *Ps. aeruginosa* is often the cause of death in CF.

4. Leukemic, transplant, or **neutropenic patients** (<500 PMNs/mm^3): **septicemia, pneumonia, or both**

5. Patients with long-term urinary catheters: UTIs

6. IV drug abusers: endocarditis, osteomyelitis, arthritis

7. Diabetics: malignant otitis externa

E. Drug resistance. *Pseudomonas* has native resistance to many antibiotics. Order susceptibility testing.

II. *LEGIONELLA*

A. Characteristics. *Legionella* is a genus of **poorly Gram staining, intracellular, aerobic bacilli.** *Legionella pneumophila* is the most common causative agent of legionnaires' disease; *Legionella micdadei* is next.

B. Reservoirs and transmission. *Legionella* is a water organism (often found intracellularly in amoebae in streams). It contaminates air conditioning systems. There is **no human-to-human transmission!**

C. Virulence factors. *Legionella* is **intracellular** in humans, landing in the alveoli; it is taken up, survives, and multiplies in the monocyte/macrophage series, ultimately killing the cells.

D. Infections. **Legionnaire's disease** is a necrotizing, multifocal pneumonia characterized by **myalgia, headache, fever, diarrhea, and initially nonproductive cough.** It is most severe in compromised patients.

E. Laboratory identification

1. **Gram stain** result is Gram-negative if counterstain time is increased.

2. **Buffered Charcoal Yeast Extract (BCYE) agar** provides cysteine and ferric iron.

III. *BORDETELLA*

A. Characteristics. *Bordetella* is a genus of small, **Gram-negative, aerobic extracellular bacilli.** *Bordetella pertussis* is the most common human pathogen. The organism is not invasive. Instead, *B. pertussis* attaches to respiratory epithelium through **filamentous hemagglutination and an adhesin called pertactin.** *Bordetella pertussis* is the most common human pathogen. The organism is not invasive.

B. Toxins are the primary mediators of infection.

1. **Pertussis toxin** is an **A-B component toxin.** The A component, an **ADP-ribosyl transferase, inhibits G_i** (i.e., it inhibits the inhibitor of adenylate cyclase); thus cAMP increases in target cells. Lymphocytosis and hypoglycemia result clinically.

2. **Adenylate cyclase** produced by *B. pertussis* enters human cells, where the intracellular calmodulin activates it to cause an increase in intracellular cAMP.

3. **Tracheal cytotoxin** inhibits respiratory epithelial cilia and ultimately kills the cells.

C. Reservoir. Humans (even vaccinated) are the only reservoir. Vaccine-induced immunity wanes at about 11 years; >20% of coughs that persist >2 weeks in afebrile adults are pertussis.

D. Infection. Pertussis follows a 7- to 10-day incubation.

1. The **catarrhal stage** lasts 1–2 weeks; the infection is contagious during this stage. Symptoms include rhinorrhea (copious and mucoid) and symptoms of a cold, but fever is generally not prominent.

2. The **paroxysmal stage** is marked by repetitive short expiratory bursts through a narrowed glottis, ending in inspiratory gasp and often vomiting. The severity of the cough in unvaccinated individuals frequently leads to aspiration pneumonia, eye hemorrhages, hernias, frenal ulcers, and seizures. In some cases there is permanent CNS damage. Lymphocytosis is common. The cough persists for 2 to 4 weeks. **Bordetellae disappear by the end of the paroxysmal stage.**

3. The **convalescent stage** includes decreased cough and recovery, unless permanent CNS damage has occurred.

E. Laboratory identification. Tests are **nasopharyngeal mucus cultures** or cough plates **on Regan-Lowe** and **direct immunofluorescence** on specimens. Cultures are generally negative (even though the person has pertussis) if antibiotics have already been used, if symptoms have been present for more than 4 weeks, or if the individual has been vaccinated. Thus, diagnosis is often clinical.

F. Prevention. All **new DTaP vaccinations** include the **pertussis filamentous hemagglutinin** and the **pertussis toxoid;** they vary in other components. Babies are born without immunity and are at extremely high risk of exposure and disease if not vaccinated.

IV. *FRANCISELLA*

A. Characteristics. *Francisella* is a genus of facultative intracellular, Gram-negative bacilli. The most important human pathogen of this genus is *Francisella tularensis.*

B. Reservoir and transmission. *F. tularensis* infects wild mammals, often without overt disease; human infections start with:

1. **Animal blood** (typically rabbits) entering a **human** via a **cut** while skinning the animal or by **inhalation** of an aerosol

2. **Bite** of an infected **tick or deer fly**

3. Ingestion of **rare meat**

C. Infections. Ulceroglandular tularemia (most common) begins with fever chills, malaise, and an ulcerating papule at the inoculation site.

D. Laboratory identification. Diagnosis is by **serology** or **immunofluorescent microscopy.** *Francisella* is **hazardous** to culture, so it is cultured only in reference labs.

V. *BRUCELLA*

A. Characteristics. *Brucella* is a genus of Gram-negative, **facultative intracellular bacilli** that localize in the cells of the **reticuloendothelial system.**

B. Reservoir and transmission. Brucellae cause **GU tract infections in goats, pigs, and cattle.** *Brucella* is spread from infected animals by **direct mucosal contact, traumatic skin implantation,** or **ingestion** and therefore is an occupational hazard of veterinarians, slaughterhouse workers, farmers, and anyone who ingests **unpasteurized dairy products,** particularly outside the U.S.

C. Infections. Brucellosis or **undulant fever** is an **influenzalike disease** that may cause temperature undulations, with **drenching sweats in late afternoon or evening.** Disease varies from mild and self-limiting (**Br. abortus** from cattle) to serious (**Br. melitensis** from goats). It may be chronic (most commonly with **Br. suis** *from swine*), may resemble chronic fatigue syndrome, and may be associated with depression that lasts for years.

D. Laboratory identification. Diagnosis is made by serology and blood cultures. **Special handling** is required; notify the lab.

13

Gram-Negative Microaerophilic Curved Bacteria

Campylobacter, Helicobacter

I. CAMPYLOBACTER

A. Characteristics. This genus consists of **Gram-negative curved** rods, each with a polar flagellum. The organisms are often found in "nose-to-nose" pairs that look like flying seagull's wings. *Campylobacter* is **microaerophilic,** fastidious (requires specific media), **grows at 42°C (107°F),** and is oxidase-positive like *Vibrio* but a nonfermenter. The most important human pathogen of this genus is ***Campylobacter jejuni.***

B. Reservoirs and transmission. *Campylobacter jejuni* exists as normal GI tract flora of many wild and domestic animals, including dogs. Human infection is most often through ingestion of raw or undercooked poultry.

C. Infection: bacterial enteritis. *Campylobacter jejuni* is one of the most common causes of infectious diarrhea (an estimated 40% of cases in U.S.). Symptoms include acute abdominal pain (sometimes resembling appendicitis), diarrhea with blood and pus, malaise, and fever. Disease is generally self-limiting, lasting <7 days.

D. Laboratory identification. Diagnosis of *Campylobacter* is by **microaerophilic culture** on special media (**Skirrow's** or Campy medium).

E. Sequelae. Arthritis or Guillain-Barré may follow in the recovery period.

II. HELICOBACTER

A. Characteristics. This genus consists of **Gram-negative,** curved bacteria, each with a tuft of polar **flagella.** *Helicobacter pylori* is the most important species to humans. It is **microaerophilic** and **urease-positive;** it survives stomach acid by creating an ammonia cloud around it. It penetrates the gastric mucous layer where it invades tissues and causes **gastritis** and **ulcers;** chronic *H. pylori* ulcers are associated with gastric carcinomas.

B. Reservoirs and transmission. Transmission is by the fecal-oral route. Gastroscopes may also spread *Helicobacter* if not properly cleaned.

C. Laboratory identification

1. Microaerophilic culture of biopsy specimen at 37°C (98.6°F).

2. Urease breath test

3. Serology for *H. pylori* antibodies

D. Treatment of infection. The most common treatment is bismuth + metronidazole + tetracycline + omeprazole.

14

Gram-Negative Facultative Anaerobic Bacilli—Family Enterobacteriaceae

Escherichia, Klebsiella, Salmonella, Shigella, Proteus, Yersinia

I. INTRODUCTION TO THE ENTEROBACTERIACEAE FAMILY*

A. Characteristics. The Enterobacteriaceae family consists of Gram-negative rods that are facultative anaerobes. **All ferment glucose** and **are oxidase-negative** and catalase-positive. **All reduce nitrates to nitrites.** High-yield genera of the Enterobacteriaceae are listed **in Table 14-1.**

B. Virulence factors: surface antigens. **Figure 14-1** is a visual memory trick of the three antigens: O, H, and K antigen. **Pili,** which aid adherence, **and outer membrane proteins** (OMPs) may also be present.

II. *ESCHERICHIA*

A. Characteristics. This genus consists of **lactose-fermenting Enterobacteriaceae.** *Escherichia coli* is the most important human pathogen of this genus. Most strains of *E. coli* are nonpathogenic, normal intestinal flora; other strains are pathogens with differing virulence factors and effects.

B. Infections

    1. UTIs. *E. coli* is the most common cause of both community-acquired and nosocomial UTI.

        a. Virulence factors. Strains causing pyelonephritis generally have either P-pili (pyelonephritis-associated pili) or x-adhesins, both of which adhere to the uroepithelium.

        b. Transmission. The infecting bacteria come from our own fecal flora.

        c. Laboratory identification. First-time UTIs are assumed to be *E. coli* and are treated empirically with trimethoprim-sulfamethoxazole without laboratory ID. Diagnostic methods include:

            (1) Dipstick tests. These show positive leukocyte esterase (sign of pus in urine, not always associated with bacteriuria), positive nitrites, and presence of Gram-negative bacteria on unspun urine.

            (2) Quantitative cultures. Counts >1,000/ml urine are now considered positive in a symptomatic individual.

---

*It is easier to learn the Enterobacteriaceae family characteristics and which organisms are Enterobacteriaceae than to learn characteristics like nitrate reduction for each genus.

Table 14-1
High-Yield Genera of the Enterobacteriaceae

Lactose fermenters = CEEK
C = *Citrobacter*
E = *Enterobacter*
E = *Escherichia*
K = *Klebsiella*

Lactose fermenters = ShYPS
Sh = *Shigella* Y = *Yersinia*	Non-motile; no H_2S produced
P = *Proteus* S = *Salmonella*	Highly motile; H_2S produced

2. Diarrheas
    a. **Enterotoxic *E. coli.*** ETEC is a major cause of **"traveler's diarrhea"** and of infant diarrhea in developing countries.
       (1) **Virulence factors** include **heat-labile toxin (LT), an A-B component toxin with ADP-ribosyl transferase activity that stimulates G_s;** this increases adenylate cyclase activity and cAMP. There is also a heat-stable toxin (ST) that turns on a guanylate cyclase. *E. coli* causes a noninvasive, watery diarrhea with abdominal cramping requiring only supportive care.

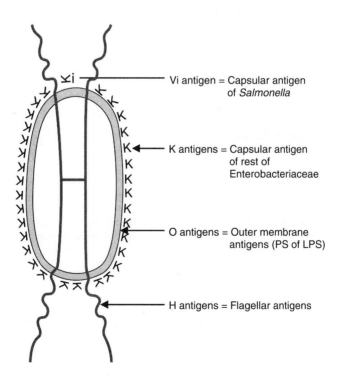

Figure 14-1. Enterobacteriaceae antigens memory trick (not diagram of structure). **O *antigens*** are the polysaccharide part of LPS in the bacterial cell envelope (the big "O" in the figure). **H *antigens*** are the flagella that are present on some Enterobacteriaceae. (You can visualize a huge letter "H" with helical ends as the flagella.) **K *antigens*** are polysaccharide capsular antigens that are present on some Enterobacteriaceae.

      (2) **Reservoir and transmission.** ETEC is transmitted in developing countries through use of human feces as fertilizer on food crops and generally poor sanitation.

    b. **Enteropathogenic *E. coli*.** EPEC is a major cause of chronic diarrhea and a reason for failure to thrive in infants in developing countries (although rotavirus is more common). EPEC is not considered invasive but adheres (**virulence factor**), causing lesions by surface effacement.

    c. **Enteroinvasive *E. coli*.** EIEC causes dysentery similar to that of shigellosis (fever, diarrhea, vomiting, abdominal cramping, and tenesmus); many patients have blood and pus in the stools, although some only have watery diarrhea. **EIEC virulence** is due to invasion of intestinal epithelium. **Transmission** may be associated with contaminated food.

    d. **Enterohemorrhagic *E. coli*.** EHEC's most common strain is O157:H7.

      (1) **Reservoir and transmission.** EHEC may be found in food contaminated by cattle feces (mainly hamburger).

      (2) **Infection and toxicities.** EHEC produces a hemorrhagic toxin called a **verotoxin,** which is **a shigalike toxin.** Clinically these infections (also called **verotoxic *E. coli*** or VTEC) are characterized by frankly bloody diarrhea (hemorrhagic colitis) and may progress to hemolytic uremic syndrome (HUS) and acute renal failure. **Antibiotics** are contraindicated; they increase the risk of kidney damage.

  3. **Neonatal septicemia** and **meningitis.** Strains of *E. coli* involved in meningitis are **K1 encapsulated strains** that are resistant to phagocytic removal from the blood stream. (Note, however, that Group B streptococci are generally more common than *E. coli* as causative agents of neonatal meningitis.)

III. KLEBSIELLA

A. **Characteristics.** This genus consists of lactose-fermenting rods. The most common species is *Klebsiella pneumoniae*.

B. **Virulence factor.** *Klebsiella's* large polysaccharide capsule is its major virulence factor.

C. **Reservoir and transmission.** *Klebsiella* is found in human upper respiratory and GI tracts. It is **opportunistic.**

D. Infections

  1. *Klebsiella* pneumonia occurs primarily in patients with underlying pulmonary disease or alcoholism. (Note, however: *Strep. pneumoniae* is the most common cause of pneumonia in alcoholics.) *K. pneumoniae* tends to cause pneumonia with difficult-to-treat abscesses and a dark-red bloody sputum (currant jelly sputum). Sputum is generally not malodorous.

  2. *Klebsiella* UTIs occur most commonly in patients with urinary catheters.

IV. SALMONELLA

A. **Characteristics.** *Salmonella*, a nonlactose fermenting genus of Enterobacteriaceae, has 1,500 different serotypes, each with its own species name (some colorful like *S. oysterbed!*). Remember, all Enterobacteriaceae are Gram-negative rods, are oxidase-negative and catalase-positive, ferment glucose, and reduce nitrates to nitrites.

B. **Virulence.** The *Salmonella* **Vi** (virulence) **antigen** is a **capsular** polysaccharide antigen. *Salmonella* is highly motile and pathogenic.

C. *Salmonella typhi*

1. **Virulence factors.** S. *typhi* attacks the ileocecal region, invading and killing M cells. Organisms are then picked up by macrophages in the Peyer's patches. The bacteria inhibit phagosomal-lysosomal fusion. The salmonellae replicate in the phagosome, kill the macrophages, and spread through the reticuloendothelial system, eventually reaching the blood stream, leaving focal lesions in about 10% of cases. Eventually, S. *typhi* in the biliary tree is carried into the intestinal tract.

2. **Reservoir and transmission.** Unlike all other species of *Salmonella*, **S. *typhi's* only reservoir is humans.** Transmission is fecal-oral. Some people are permanent carriers.

3. **Infections. Typhoid** symptoms include gradual onset of headache, loss of appetite, malaise, lethargy, and fever, with abdominal pain and constipation early, followed by diarrhea after the second week. Fever (up to 40°C [104°F]) and bacteremia may last several weeks. Hepatosplenomegaly and mesenteric lymphadenopathy are common. Rose spots appear on the abdomen in about 25% of cases, and focal lesions occur in the very young or old.

4. **Laboratory identification.** Early diagnosis is made by blood culture; later diagnosis is made by blood, fecal, urine cultures or **Widal test** for patient antibodies to O and H antigens.

5. **Treatment** may be complicated with shock.

D. *Salmonella enteritidis* and other *Salmonella* species

1. **Reservoir and transmission.** There are many animal reservoirs; transmission is mainly from raw poultry or eggs, reptilian pets, or raw milk. Studies of milk have shown the infectious dose (30% or ID_{30}) to be 10^5 organisms in people with normal stomach acid. The very young or very old are most likely to develop disease and to have serious disease. There is high potential for spread within families.

2. Infections
   a. **Gastroenteritis.** *Salmonella* is invasive, causing fever and producing an inflammatory but watery diarrhea with abdominal pain, some nausea, and vomiting; however, it is generally self-limiting. S. *enteritidis* generally does not invade vasculature to cause septicemias, so focal lesions (seen at times with S. *cholera-suis* or S. *dublin*) are rare except in sickle cell disease. Most salmonellae are resistant to serum killing.
   b. **Osteomyelitis in sickle cell disease (SCD) patients (not carriers).** Due to functional asplenism and defective opsonic activity and alternate complement pathways, SCD patients have repeated infections with encapsulated organisms and extremely high rates of osteomyelitis. **In SCD, *Salmonella enteritidis* is the most common (>80%) causative agent of osteomyelitis.** (S. *aureus*, the most common in all other patients, rarely has a capsule.)

V. *SHIGELLA*

A. **Characteristics.** *Shigella* consists of Gram-negative rods that ferment glucose, reduce nitrates to nitrites, are oxidase-negative and catalase-positive (Guess what family!), and do little else (don't ferment lactose, don't make hydrogen sulfide, and are not motile). The most common species in the U.S. are **Sh. *sonnei*** and **Sh. *flexneri*;** the most severe is **Sh. *dysenteriae*** (rare in U.S.).

B. Virulence factors

1. *Shigella* **invades through M intestinal epithelial cells.** Polymerization of actin tails helps *Shigella* (like *Listeria*) move laterally into adjoining epithelial cells, creating

the very characteristic shallow *Shigella* ulcers without vascular invasion; thus bacteremia is rare.

    2. Shiga toxin. Type 1 strains of *Sh. dysenteriae* cause the most severe disease because they invade and produce shiga toxin (an A-B component toxin), which **cleaves the 60S ribosomal rRNA,** inhibiting protein synthesis. Shiga toxin has neurotoxic, cytotoxic, and enterotoxic effects.

C. Reservoir and transmission. The reservoir for shigellae is **humans;** spread is fecal-oral.

D. Infections. Shigellosis symptoms vary widely depending on the nutritional status and age of the patient, the infective strain, and the dose. Most cases are self-limiting. Classically, symptoms include **fever, tenesmus, frequent low-volume stools with both blood and pus present, and abdominal cramping.**

E. Laboratory identification. Diagnosis is made by **culture** on media (MacConkey and a specialized medium like *Salmonella/Shigella* agar), and by **methylene blue stain** of mucus from stools, which shows many PMNs.

VI. *PROTEUS*

A. Characteristics. *Proteus* spp. are Enterobacteriaceae noted for swarming motility and urease production. *Proteus vulgaris* and *Proteus mirabilis* are common.

B. Virulence factors. *Proteus* increases pH by **urease production,** and thus in UTIs may cause production of **renal calculi; motility** may aid entry to the bladder.

C. Reservoirs of *Proteus* are water and human feces.

D. Infections. *Proteus mirabilis* causes UTIs, and *Proteus vulgaris* is an important nosocomial opportunist.

VII. *YERSINIA*

A. *Yersinia pestis*

    1. Characteristics. This species of coagulase-positive Enterobacteriaceae is facultative intracellular with bipolar staining.

    2. Virulence factors. The important antigens are V and W and an envelope antigen, F-1, which protects against phagocytosis; endotoxin is present.

    3. Reservoir and transmission. In the U.S., the reservoir is wild rodents in the desert of the Southwest. *Y. pestis* is transmitted by:
        a. Flea bites. Infected flea feeds on a human.
        b. Respiratory droplet from human cases with pneumonic plague. (All patients should be considered **highly infectious** by respiratory route until after 72 hours of effective antibiotic therapy.)

    4. Infection: Bubonic plague. Symptoms include rapidly enlarging buboes (lymph nodes), fever, and conjunctivitis. Gram-negative septicemia may lead to pulmonary emboli, pneumonic plague (highly contagious), and shock with DIC. Fatality rate is high (>50%) if untreated.

    5. Prevention and treatment. The patient is put in isolation for 72 hours after antibiotics are started. Because *Y. pestis* is facultative intracellular, antibiotics used must be those that penetrate eukaryotic cells well and are effective against Gram-negative cells: generally gentamicin, streptomycin, or doxycycline.

B. *Yersinia enterocolitica*

1. Characteristics. Like *Listeria monocytogenes*, *Y. enterocolitica* is a zoonotic, GI tract organism that can grow in cold.

2. Reservoirs and transmission. *Y. enterocolitica* is transmitted by direct contact or in food products such as raw milk.

3. Infection: Invasive enterocolitis. Symptoms include blood and pus in diarrhea, fever, symptoms of appendicitis, or reactive polyarthritis. Because *Y. enterocolitica* grows under refrigeration, it may cause blood transfusion-associated infections.

VIII. OTHER ENTEROBACTERIACEAE. Other genera of the Enterobacteriaceae family are seen as infective agents mainly in compromised or hospitalized patients. Those causing septicemias include *Enterobacter, Citrobacter, Arizona, Providencia, Morganella,* and *Serratia* (noted for its salmon-red pigment).

15

Gram-Negative Facultative Anaerobic Bacilli (Non-Enterobacteriaceae)

Vibrio, Haemophilus, Pasteurella

I. *VIBRIO.* Vibrios are **comma-shaped** bacilli with one polar flagellum. Vibrios are facultative anaerobes but, unlike the Enterobacteriaceae, are **oxidase-positive.**

A. *Vibrio cholerae*

1. **Characteristics. *Vibrio cholerae*** is noninvasive and prefers an alkaline environment. O1 strains of the El Tor biotype of *Vibrio cholerae* are the most frequent causative agents of cholera.

2. **Reservoir and transmission.** *V. cholerae* is transmitted by **human fecal contamination of water and food** including shellfish from contaminated waters. The infective dose is high, about 10^7 *if* stomach acid is normal.

3. **Virulence factors.** Cholera toxin **binds to GM1-ganglioside receptors;** the internalized A component ADP-ribosylates G_s, persistently stimulating G_s, resulting in **high cAMP levels** and **active efflux of ions and water into lumen of the small intestine.**

4. **Infection: Cholera.** *Vibrio cholerae* strains cause a **dramatic watery diarrhea ("rice-water stools")** in which fluid loss is so great that **hypovolemic shock** will occur if electrolytes and fluids are not replaced. There may be vomiting, but there is no fever or blood or pus in stools. After recovery, there is a long lasting immunity.

5. **Laboratory identification.** A **special alkaline medium, TCBS** (thiosulfate citrate-bile salts-sucrose), enhances growth. (Learn only the TCBS and alkaline medium.)

6. **Treatment.** Fluid and electrolytes are critical. Ciprofloxacin or norfloxacin reduces carriage and shortens the duration of illness.

B. *Vibrio parahaemolyticus*

1. **Reservoir and transmission. *V. parahaemolyticus*** is a coastal marine saltwater **(halophilic)** species that infects humans through **undercooked or raw sea food.**

2. **Disease.** *V. parahaemolyticus* **gastroenteritis** is characterized by a **self-limiting, explosive, watery diarrhea, vomiting, and fever.**

C. *Vibrio vulnificus*

1. **Reservoir and transmission.** *V. vulnificus* is also halophilic, contaminating oysters. In the U.S., some oyster beds along the Gulf of Mexico coast have been implicated.

2. **Diseases: Cellulitis, gastroenteritis, and septicemia.** A serious necrotic cellulitis occurs in cuts (from shucking contaminated oysters). **Ingestion of raw contami-**

nated oysters causes a gastroenteritis and, in patients with liver or iron-overload conditions, it may also cause septicemia and death.

II. HAEMOPHILUS

A. Characteristics. Haemophili are Gram-negative pleomorphic* rods. These bacteria are fastidious, requiring growth factors from lysed blood (*Haemophilus* means **"heme-loving"**). There are two important genera for humans: *H. influenzae and H. ducreyi.*

B. *Haemophilus influenzae* (H. *flu*)

   1. Virulence factors. The major factor is the **polyribitol type B capsule.** Nonencapsulated forms are part of our normal nasopharyngeal flora; encapsulated ("typeable") strains cause a variety of illnesses, with strain B being the most common.

   2. Infections and toxicities

   a. Otitis media, sinusitis, and **bronchitis** are caused primarily by **nontypeable strains of H. *flu.***

   b. Septicemia is caused by encapsulated forms (most commonly type B) that colonize upper respiratory tract mucosa and infect unvaccinated children ages 6 months to 2 years.

   c. Purulent epidemic meningitis occurs when *H. influenzae* crosses the blood-brain barrier during septicemia in susceptible babies. Because of high vaccination rates in this country, *H. flu* is no longer the most common cause of meningitis in children under 2 years of age. (*N. meningitidis* is more common.)

   d. Epiglottitis is usually caused by type B *H. influenzae*. It occurs most often in 2- to 4-year-old boys. Symptoms are **fever, dysphagia, drooling, sore throat, inspiratory stridor, and cherry red epiglottis** protruding into the airway. The child will often want to sit hunched over and not lie down. Maintenance of airway and administration of antibiotics are important. There has been a dramatic decrease in cases due to vaccination.

   3. Laboratory identification

   a. Chocolate agar (a lysed blood agar) provides both the **X (protoporphyrin)** and the **V (NAD) factors** that are required for growth.

   b. On **blood agar,** *H. influenzae* grows around *Staphylococcus aureus*; this "**satellite phenomenon**" occurs because *Staphylococcus* produces NAD and lyses erythrocytes.

   4. Prevention. Vaccination with B capsular polysaccharide, which is complexed to protein, prevents *H. flu* type B disease.

C. *Haemophilus influenzae* var. *aegypticus* causes **bacterial pink eye,** which has a **purulent** discharge.

D. *Haemophilus ducreyi* is a species that is more common in the tropics and in the southern U.S. It causes **chancroid,** a sexually transmitted disease (STD) characterized by **painful genital ulcers.** (🔊 You do cry with *ducreyi.*) Chancroid lesions heal slowly and may increase the risk of HIV transmission. There now is a polymerase chain reaction (PCR) test to identify *H. ducreyi.*

III. PASTEURELLA. This genus consists of organisms that are **normal oral flora in many animals. *Pasteurella multocida*** is transmitted by **dog, pig, and cat bites** (domestic house cats or lions). Cat bites in particular need to be treated; amoxicillin + clavulanate is the treatment of choice.

---

*Pleomorphic** means variable in morphology. For instance, encapsulated *H. influenzae* from CSF are short coccobacilli, but nonencapsulated forms found in ear infections may be nearly filamentous.

16

Gram-Negative Anaerobic Bacilli and Cocci

Bacteroides, Prevotella/Porphyromonas, Fusobacterium

I. GENERAL NOTES

   A. **Reservoirs.** Most medically important anaerobic Gram-negative bacteria are **opportunists found in the normal flora of the upper respiratory tract, mouth, colon, and female genital tract.**

   B. **Infections.** These bacteria cause **endogenous,** mixed infections (autoinfection), commonly when they enter normally sterile devitalized tissues or create anaerobic fluid pockets (**empyema**). They are major causative agents of **empyema** or **abscesses** in respiratory, intestinal, or genital tracts or bone or soft tissue. Anaerobes play a role in **chronic otitis media and sinusitis,** aspiration pneumonia (foul smelling sputum), and also in infections in **diabetic patients** such as **decubitus ulcers.**

   C. **Laboratory identification. Specimens must be taken and transported anaerobically** (and quickly) to the lab for **anaerobic culture.**

   D. **Species.** You do not need species-specific information, except that *Bacteroides fragilis* is the **most common bacterium** in your body.

II. *BACTEROIDES.* This genus consists of thin, Gram-negative bacilli. *Bacteroides fragilis* is aerotolerant (so is really *not* fragile) and is the most common fecal microorganism. The **capsule** of *B. fragilis* is **antiphagocytic** and **stimulates abscess** formation. The **modified *Bacteroides* endotoxin** has reduced toxicity.

III. *PREVOTELLA/PORPHYROMONAS.* *Prevotella/Porphyromonas* complex is normal oral and genital flora that is noted for **pigment** production. (*Prevotella melaninogenica* was formerly known as *Bacteroides melaninogenicus.* The USMLE Step 1 will probably give you both names.) Infections with *Prevotella/Porphyromonas* include oral (and human bite), respiratory, and GU tract infections and are **difficult to treat,** requiring debridement as well as antibiotics.

IV. *FUSOBACTERIUM.* Fusobacteria are Gram-negative anaerobes, slender cells with tapered, pointed ends. In addition to playing a role in some of the infections described above, *Fusobacterium,* along with spirochetal oral flora, **overgrows** to cause ulcerative oral-pharyngeal lesions called **Vincent's angina.**

17

Spirochetes (Gram-Negative Envelope)

Treponema, Borrelia, Leptospira

I. GENERAL CHARACTERISTICS. Spirochetes are Gram-negative, spiral-shaped bacteria so thin that they **do not show up well with light microscopy** (e.g., Gram stain) even though they have Gram-negative peptidoglycan and an outer membrane with endotoxin. The cell is held in its spiral shape by an "internal" flagellum (immediately under the outer membrane). This **axial filament** is attached at each end, producing a distinctive **springing motility.** Spirochetes are best visualized by dark field or fluorescent microscopy.

II. *TREPONEMA*

A. Characteristics. This genus consists of some microaerophilic, extracellular organisms. Pathogenic strains are not routinely cultured on inert media. *T. pallidum* is the major pathogen in the U.S. It is **easily visualized by darkfield microscopy** from the primary chancre or from secondary mucous membrane lesions.

B. Reservoir and transmission. Humans are the only significant reservoir for *T. pallidum*, which is transmitted through sexual contact or across the placenta.

C. Infection. Syphilis (untreated) is a **multistage disease.** Many features of syphilis are attributed to blood vessel involvement. The **incubation period** is variable, generally **about 3 weeks.** The following description is the potential development in untreated syphilis.

1. Primary syphilis consists of a nontender, indurated ulcer (chancre) with fairly smooth margins at the site of inoculation, with early bacteremia and spread to regional lymph nodes. Chancres are **highly infectious** but heal spontaneously in 3 to 6 weeks.

2. Secondary syphilis appears 1 to 3 months later. *T. pallidum* spreads via the blood stream, producing flulike disease with **infectious flat, hyperpigmented rash** on the skin, and **infectious, moist, papular lesions** on the mucous membranes. It may spread to any organ. Secondary syphilis may also "heal" spontaneously.

3. The **latent stage** may be interrupted by relapses of secondary syphilis and then become truly latent.

4. Tertiary syphilis may appear decades after the primary infection if untreated. **Aortitis** is characteristic, along with variable **CNS involvement** (neurosyphilis) or gummas in bones, skin, or viscera.

5. Congenital syphilis. *T. pallidum* crosses the placenta. Congenital syphilis symptoms range from **stillbirths** to **multiple fetal abnormalities,** or babies may be asymptomatic until the age of 2 to 5 years.

D. Laboratory identification. *T. pallidum* is not routinely cultured. Diagnosis is based on microscopy (material from lesions) or clinical presentation and serology.

1. **Microscopy.** *T. pallidum* is too thin to be seen by light microscopy, so **darkfield** or **direct fluorescent antibody** is used **(Fig.17–1).** Specimen sources include chancres, secondary mucous membrane lesions, lymph nodes, and tissues.

2. **Serologic tests.** Two different antibodies are made in response to syphilis. The **earliest** antibody is **antitreponemal antibody,** which binds to treponemes. Approximately one week later, **nontreponemal antibody (reagin)** appears. This nonspecific antibody appears to be stimulated by cellular damage. Nontreponemal antibody binds to mammalian cardiolipid (a very cheap antigen) but not to treponemes. These two antibodies are detected in the serological diagnostic tests

   a. **Nontreponemal (reaginic) tests** are inexpensive screening tests, because the antigen is cow heart cardiolipin-lecithin, which detects only patient reaginic antibody. Nontreponemal tests have high sensitivity (detect most cases) but low specificity (detect other diseases too, but not usually other spirochetes). **Nontreponemal antibody titers decrease** with antibiotic treatment or **spontaneously in late latent phase. Nontreponemal tests** include:

      (1) VDRL (Venereal Disease Research Laboratory test)
      (2) RPR (rapid plasma reagin test)
      (3) ART (automated reagin test)

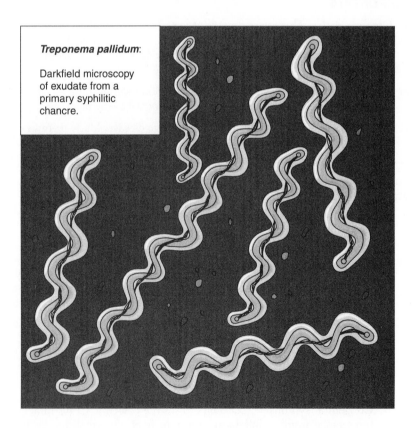

Treponema pallidum:

Darkfield microscopy of exudate from a primary syphilitic chancre.

Figure 17-1. *T. pallidum* is seen in a "negative" pattern on darkfield microscopy.

b. **Treponemal antibody tests** use expensive treponemal antigens and thus **detect specific treponemal antibody.** These expensive tests are used to confirm all positive nontreponemal screening tests. These tests have high sensitivity and better specificity (**except** that they may be positive in any spirochete disease such as Lyme disease). Antitreponemal antibody titer increases with infection and remains positive for many years, even with treatment. **Common treponemal tests** include:

(1) **FTAB-ABS** (fluorescent treponemal antibody-absorption test)

(2) **MHA-TP** (microhemagglutination-*Treponema pallidum* test)

E. **Treatment of infection.** Treatment of primary or secondary syphilis infections is **benzathine penicillin.**

III. **BORRELIA** are larger and more loosely coiled spirochetes than treponemes. Known pathogenic species are arthropod-borne.

A. *Borrelia burgdorferi*

1. **Virulence factors.** *Borrelia burgdorferi* may be **intracellular;** thus polymerase chain reaction (PCR) from body fluids may not be positive. The organism may access immunologically privileged sites like CNS, tendons, vitreous humor, and synoviae. There is evidence of antigenic variation.

2. **Reservoir and transmission.** Reservoirs are white-footed **mice** and white-tailed **deer.** Vectors are *Ixodes* **ticks** (a.k.a. black-legged or deer ticks). Any stage of the tick can carry the infection, but nymphs (< 0.5 mm) are the most common vector. *Ixodes scapularis* (formerly *I. dammini*) is the vector in northeast and north central U.S., and *Ixodes pacificus* the vector in western U.S.

3. **Infection: Lyme disease (LD).** Infection starts with an infecting **deer tick bite. Initial clinical symptoms** may include erythema (chronicum) migrans (EM), the spreading erythematous **"target" lesion,** as well as fever, chills, fatigue, headache, and muscle or joint pain. **Dissemination** may occur as early as days to weeks later; multiple symptoms develop and may include **multiple EM, Bell's palsy, fever, stiff neck, headache, limb numbness or pain,** arrhythmias, persistent malaise, and fatigue. **Late symptoms** (polyarthritis, neurologic impairment, and fatigue) may develop months to years later if the primary disease is not treated successfully. Patients may have mixed infections with *Borrelia*, *Ehrlichia*, or *Babesia*. Congenital infections occur. Reinfections may occur.

4. **Laboratory identification.** *Borrelia* are Gram-negative but are not seen well in Gram stains. **Diagnosis** is done by serology, PCR, microscopy (using acridine orange), or culture (modified Kelly medium). There are false negative serologies due to intracellular sequestering of organisms, heavy antigenic load (so no free antibody), antigenic variation of causative strains, and so on.

5. **Treatment** depends on the stage of the infection.

B. *Borrelia recurrentis* and other *Borrelia* spp.

1. **Reservoir and transmission.** *Borrelia recurrentis* is louse-borne. Other *Borrelia* infections are tick-borne.

2. **Infections. Relapsing fever** is characterized by an abrupt onset of symptoms: shaking chills, fever, muscle aches, headache, delirium, cough, lethargy, splenomegaly, and hepatomegaly. This is followed by spontaneous resolution of symptoms. Symptoms recur and resolve again about a week later, then recur less severely and resolve one more time. **Antigenic phase variation** is responsible for recurring septicemias.

3. **Laboratory identification.** Diagnosis is by Giemsa stain.

IV. *LEPTOSPIRA*

A. Characteristics. Leptospires are fine spirochetes with hooked ends. The most important species is *Leptospira interrogans*.

B. Reservoir and transmission. Leptospires are found in a variety of wild and domestic animals and are transferred by **animal urine in water.** In the U.S. the organism is generally transferred by contact with dog, livestock, or rat urine (e.g., while working in sewers), by puddle stomping, or by recreation in contaminated water.

C. Infection. Leptospirosis generally presents like influenza with or without abdominal pain, vomiting, and conjunctival suffusion. If untreated, it may progress to hepatitis, renal failure, and aseptic meningitis.

D. Laboratory identification. Identification of this organism requires special procedures. Notify the lab.

18

Rickettsiaceae (Gram-Negative Envelope)

Rickettsia, Coxiella, Bartonella, Ehrlichia

I. **GENERAL CHARACTERISTICS.** The Rickettsiaceae family includes the genera *Rickettsia, Coxiella, Bartonella* (formerly known as *Rochalimaea*), and *Ehrlichia*. All but *Bartonella* are obligate intracellular parasites that make limited ATP. They have a Gram-negative cell envelope but are not seen well on Gram stain because of their small size. **Known vectors and reservoir hosts for each rickettsia and disease** are shown in **Table 18-1.** Where you need to know more than the vector and reservoir hosts, additional information is given in the text.

II. ***RICKETTSIA*** (*Rickettsia rickettsii*)

 A. **Characteristics.** *Rickettsia rickettsii* (⬤ the "double-named" rickettsia) causes the most important rickettsial disease in the U.S., Rocky Mountain spotted fever **(RMSF).** It is an obligate intracellular pathogen.

 B. **Reservoir and transmission.** Reservoir **hosts** are **rodents, dogs,** and *Dermacentor* **ticks.** (The **ticks** are **reservoirs** because of transovarian transmission.) **Vectors** are *Dermacentor americanus* (dog) and *Amblyomma americanum* (Lone Star) ticks. Despite its name, it now occurs most commonly on the East coast of the U.S.

 C. **Infection. Rocky Mountain spotted fever (RMSF)** generally occurs in the summer, starting with a tick bite. *R. rickettsii* invades the endothelial lining of capillaries, causing vasculitis. Symptoms include abrupt onset of high fever, chills, headache, myalgia, nausea, and vomiting. A macular rash and swelling start several days later on the ankles and wrists and spread to the trunk, palms, soles, and face. Mortality is 3%.

 D. **Laboratory identification.** Diagnosis of RMSF is by immunofluorescent stain of skin biopsy or by **serology.** The old Weil-Felix test is based on the cross-reaction of *Rickettsia rickettsii* antibodies with OX strains of *P. vulgaris. Note:* culturing *R. rickettsii* (done on tissue culture) is **extremely hazardous.**

 E. **Treatment of infection. Doxycycline** (which penetrates human cells well to kill the rickettsias) is started quickly if RMSF is suspected).

III. ***COXIELLA***

 A. **Characteristics.** Like *Rickettsia* and *Ehrlichia*, the genus *Coxiella* consists of **obligate intracellular** organisms. **Coxiella burnetii** is the most significant species.

 B. **Virulence factors.** *Coxiella burnetii* is resistant to drying and can survive in the environment. This bacterium survives intracellularly by growing in phagolysosomes at low pH despite the presence of lysosomal enzymes.

Table 18-1
Rickettsial Diseases, Organisms, Vectors or Means of Transmission, and Reservoirs

Disease	Organism	Vector or Means of Transmission	Reservoir
Rickettsial diseases with rash			
Rocky Mountain spotted fever* (rash starts distal, moves to trunk)	*Rickettsia rickettsii*	Tick	Wild rodents, dogs, **ticks also reservoir**
Rickettsialpox (lesions often mistaken for chicken pox)	*Rickettsia akari*	Mite	Rodents; usually in rodent-infested housing
Trench fever (transient rash)	*Bartonella quintana*	Human body louse	Humans
Epidemic typhus (rash mainly on trunk)	*Rickettsia prowazekii*	Human body louse	Humans
Rickettsial diseases generally with no rash			
Ehrlichiosis (infection of monocytes or granulocytes)	*Ehrlichia chaffeensis* *Ehrlichia equi*	Tick	Unknown
Cat scratch fever	*Bartonella henselae*	Scratch	Kittens
Bacillary angiomatosis and septicemia	*Bartonella quintana*	Human body louse	Humans
Q fever*	*Coxiella burnetii*	Aerosols or dust inhalation; no vector**	Cattle, sheep, goats

*RMSF and Q fever are currently the most important rickettsial diseases in the U.S., but ehrlichiosis and bartonellosis are gaining importance.
**No significant arthropod vector in human disease.

C. **Reservoir and transmission.** *C. burnettii's* reservoir is domestic livestock (particularly sheep), reaching high titers in pregnant animals. Transmission is by inhalation of dust or aerosols of urine, feces, amniotic fluid, or placental tissue.

D. **Infection: Q fever.** Symptoms include **fever,** headache, chills, and atypical **(patchy interstitial) pneumonia** with a mild **dry hack. Hepatitis** often occurs. There is **NO RASH.**

E. **Laboratory identification.** Diagnosis is made by any of a number of serologic tests; Weil-Felix is negative. *Coxiella* is not seen well on Gram stain smear because it is very small. Specimens are **hazardous;** notify the lab.

IV. *BARTONELLA* (Rochalimaea)

A. **Characteristics.** Bartonellae are **pericellular,** not intracellular, rickettsias. The two significant species are **B. quintana** and **B. henselae.**

B. Infections

  1. **Trench fever,** caused by *B. quintana*, occurs in humans only; the vector is the human body louse; there were about 1 million cases in World War I.

  2. **Septicemia** with *B. henselae* is seen in homeless, HIV-negative, inner-city alcoholics. The **vector** is unknown. **Diagnosis** is by symptoms (fever with or without rash) and positive blood cultures. Endocarditis occurs in 20% of cases.

  3. In **bacillary angiomatosis** (*B. henselae*), vascular nodules develop in HIV-positive individuals.

  4. **Cat scratch fever** is caused by *B. henselae*. The organism is transmitted from an infected cat.

V. *EHRLICHIA.* Ehrlichiae infect human monocytes or granulocytes and are seen in them as mulberry-like clusters called **morulae. Ehrlichioses** are nonspecific febrile illnesses similar to **RMSF minus the rash,** but with **leukopenia** and **thrombocytopenia.** Ehrlichiosis is transmitted by ticks, so coinfections with *Borrelia burgdorferi* or *Babesia* may occur.

19

Chlamydiae
(Modified Gram-Negative Envelope)

Chlamydia

I. GENERAL CHARACTERISTICS

A. Chlamydiae are obligate intracellular bacteria that cannot make ATP. Chlamydiae have only a thin layer of **modified peptidoglycan (missing muramic acid)** between the outer and the inner membranes. They are not seen well on Gram stain.

B. Chlamydiae have a **complex life cycle:**

1. The **infectious, extracellular (⑩ out in the "elements") form** is called the **elementary body (Fig. 19-1),** which is resistant to drying, metabolically inactive, *and* has ligands to bind to epithelial cell receptors, stimulating endocytic uptake.

2. The **intracellular form** is known as the **reticulate body.** Intracellularly, elementary bodies develop into **metabolically active, dividing** reticulate bodies that produce new elementary bodies. Aggregates of reticulate bodies (**inclusion bodies**) can be visualized with fluorescent-antibody stains.

II. VIRULENCE.
All chlamydiae invade epithelium. Damage results from granuloma formation, which may lead to serotype-specific consequences, such as fallopian tube blockage (D-H), corneal scarring (A, B, Ba, C), lymphatic blockage (L1, L2, L3), and so on.

III. *CHLAMYDIA TRACHOMATIS.*
Chl. trachomatis, the major chlamydial pathogen, is sensitive to sulfonamides, and stains with iodine (because of glycogen in inclusion bodies). There are **three serotypes,** each group with distinctive epidemiology and disease patterns.

A. Serotypes D-K, common in the U.S., cause reproductive tract infections, pneumonia, and inclusion conjunctivitis.

1. **Infection in adults, especially young sexually active adults.** *Chl. trachomatis* serotypes D-K are transmitted **sexually** or by other direct contact. Infections are often subclinical, but may still cause significant fallopian tube damage. Repeated infections may occur; infertility increases to 50% with 3 or more infections. Chlamydial genital infections (about 5×10^5/year) are more common than gonorrhea (about 3×10^5/year).

2. **Infections in neonates (acquired during delivery)**

a. **Chlamydial inclusion conjunctivitis.** Infection is mucopurulent with onset of symptoms in the neonate between days 8 and 10. Erythromycin eye ointment

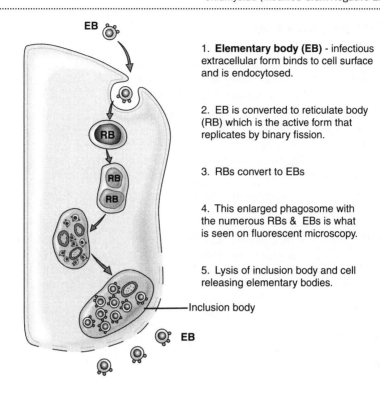

EB

1. **Elementary body (EB)** - infectious extracellular form binds to cell surface and is endocytosed.

2. EB is converted to reticulate body (RB) which is the active form that replicates by binary fission.

3. RBs convert to EBs

4. This enlarged phagosome with the numerous RBs & EBs is what is seen on fluorescent microscopy.

5. Lysis of inclusion body and cell releasing elementary bodies.

Inclusion body

EB

Figure 19-1. Life cycle of Chlamydiae.

(used at birth to prevent *N. gonorrhoeae* infection) does not prevent chlamydial conjunctivitis. Systemic erythromycin must be used to treat the eye infection and prevent chlamydial pneumonia.

b. Chlamydial pneumonia. Onset generally occurs from 2 or 3 weeks after birth to 6 months of age. Symptoms start with rhinitis and develop into a distinctive **staccato cough.** Babies are often afebrile but have difficulty feeding.

3. Laboratory identification. Nucleic acid amplification or probe tests are used for genital specimens. Inclusion bodies may be identified from direct specimens or tissue cultures with fluorescent antibody (or iodine) staining. Cultures, when done, are grown in McCoy cells.

B. Serotypes A, B, Ba, and C cause **trachoma,** a **major cause of blindness** in Asia and Africa (10 to 20 million people). Trachoma is also endemic among Native Americans in the southwestern U.S. In trachoma, chlamydiae invade the epithelium of the conjunctiva, causing **chronic follicular keratoconjunctivitis.** Follicular scarring leads to inturned eyelashes, corneal scarring and, ultimately, blindness.

C. Serotypes L1, L2, and L3 cause **lymphogranuloma venereum.** This STD, prevalent in Africa, Asia, and South America, presents with a painless **primary lesion,** fever, headache, and myalgia. **Secondary symptoms** include inflammation and swelling of lymph nodes, with systemic spread. **Tertiary symptoms** are ulcers, fistulas, and **genital elephantiasis.**

IV. *CHLAMYDIA PSITTACI*

   A. Reservoir and transmission. This zoonotic species of *Chlamydia* consists of **obligate intracellular parasites** that invade respiratory epithelium to cause **pneumonia** in **birds** (pet birds, zoo birds, turkey flocks) and humans. Transmission to humans is by exposure to an infected bird or dried bird excrement.

   B. Infection. Psittacosis is an atypical pneumonia. **Early symptoms** include headache, high fever and chills, malaise, anorexia, myalgia, arthralgia, and pale macular rash. (Remember, these are Gram-negative bacteria.) **Pulmonary symptoms** are a nonproductive cough, rales, and consolidation. **CNS involvement** is common, generally manifesting as headache, but in severe cases, encephalitis.

   C. Laboratory identification. *Chl. psittaci* is diagnosed commonly by serology; it is not seen with iodine staining.

V. *CHLAMYDIA PNEUMONIAE*. *Chl. pneumoniae* is a human pathogen spread by respiratory droplets. *Chl. pneumoniae* infection is **common but generally not severe.** Symptoms include **bronchitis, pneumonia, or sinusitis.** There are an estimated 200,000 to 300,000 cases per year, mainly in adults 18 to 45 years of age. *Chl. pneumoniae* may be associated with atherosclerosis. Laboratory identification, when needed, is by serology. **Treatment,** when needed, is generally with azithromycin.

///
Viruses

20

Viral Basics

I. EXAM STRATEGIES.
Viruses are important on the USMLE Step 1 exam. Once you understand the large concepts of **infectivity, replication,** and the **three major groups** of viruses, learn which **families** belong to each group (mnemonics help) and which **viruses** belong to which family. Then, learn the **basic diseases caused by viruses.** Most questions start with a clinical scenario requiring you to recognize the disease and know the causative agent, but often they then ask basic science questions (e.g., about replication intermediate or alcohol susceptibility), which you should be able to answer if you use the above strategy.

II. VIRAL STRUCTURE.[1]
Viruses are **acellular, obligate intracellular organisms.**

A. **Virions** are the **mature, released viruses** that can infect and take over the machinery of a host cell to make more virus.

B. **Viral genomes** are **either** DNA **or** RNA. The nucleic acid (NA) codes for all viral enzymes and structural components, except for the host-derived membrane of enveloped viruses. Some RNA viruses have more than one viral chromosome; HIV is diploid (two identical chromosomes). Others, like influenza, are segmented (more than one different chromosome).

C. **Virion proteins** include:

1. **Structural proteins** (e.g., the capsomers making up the virus "head" or **capsid**).

2. **Enzymes.** All negative ($-$) RNA viruses plus the retroviruses, hepatitis B virus, and Poxviridae have a **polymerase protein in the virion** without which they would not be able to replicate.

D. **Genomic nucleic acid + proteins** = viral **nucleocapsid.** Nucleocapsids may be **icosahedral** or **helical.**

E. **Viruses may be naked or enveloped,** as shown in **Figure 20-1.** Three of the most tested concepts are illustrated here.

1. **Naked viruses** have no lipid envelope and are all **icosahedral nucleocapsid viruses,** tightly constructed, not easily damaged by organic solvents, and more resistant to killing by chlorination. Naked viruses are released when they cause the host cells to lyse; thus, they do not cause persistent productive infections. Viral families that are naked are: Parvoviridae, Adenoviridae, and **P**apovaviridae (all DNA); **Pi**cornaviridae and **C**aliciviridae (RNA); and the dsRNA **Reo**viridae. ⦿ The naked "PAP PiCs Reo." No negative ss RNA virus is naked.

---

[1]The abbreviations **ss** for single stranded and **ds** for double stranded will be used in the following five chapters.

2. Enveloped viruses direct synthesis of specific **viral glycoproteins** that are inserted into their host's membrane. The **virus buds out** of the cell, taking on the modified host's membrane as an envelope. This "budding" type of viral release does not kill the cells outright. Thus, some enveloped viruses can set up a chronic infection.

F. Host cell range (e.g., what type of animal is infected and what tissues are infected within that host) **is determined by specific surface proteins** on each virus, which must bind to specific cellular receptors.

1. Naked icosahedral viruses bind to cell receptors through **specific surface proteins** of the capsid.

2. Enveloped viruses bind to specific host cell receptors through **viral glycoproteins embedded in an envelope. Organic solvents inactivate enveloped viruses** by damaging the lipid envelope, causing the glycoproteins that are critical for cell binding to "fall off." (There are no backup cell-binding ligands on the nucleocapsids underneath the envelope.)

Virion (Mature Virus) Structure

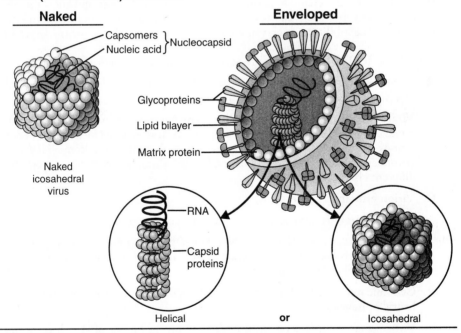

Critical concepts:
1. Surface groups (glycoproteins embedded in the lipid bilayer of the enveloped viruses or surface capsid proteins of naked capsid viruses) bind to specific host cell receptors inducing uptake, thus determining host specificity and tissue tropism.
2. The nucleic acid directs the production of the next generation of virus.
3. Some viruses (e.g., all negative RNA viruses) require a virion-associated polymerase (the actual protein in the nucleocapsid) to be infectious.

Figure 20-1.   Virion (the mature virus) structure.

III. VIRAL REPLICATION. Viruses take over their host cells and then use both host- and virus-specified components to make more virus. Steps in a generalized infection, including the **eclipse** and the **latent** periods, are shown in **Figure 20-2.** The **one-step growth curve** shown in **Figure 20-3** has been critical to our basic understanding of viral replication and is used to test your knowledge. When this test was first run, only intact virus could be detected. The diagram is highly generalized. You must be able to identify the **eclipse, latent,** and **intracellular accumulation periods,** which are labeled in the legend.

A. **Infection** takes place through **viral binding** to specific receptors (ligands) on the cell membrane, which stimulates the **uptake of the virus** through either:

1. **Fusion** of the membrane with the viral envelope (HIV, Poxviridae, or Herpesviridae).

2. Stimulation of **pinocytosis** (all naked viruses).

B. **Early macromolecular synthesis.** Once inside the cell, the viral nucleic acid is released and migrates to where it will ultimately be duplicated. The **first critical function is to produce early mRNA** in order to make early proteins. **Figure 20-4** shows how each major type of virus produces early mRNA.

C. **Replication of genome.** After early proteins are made, the virus can take over and replicate its own genome. The **nucleic acid of the progeny** virus will be **identical to that of the parent** with the **exception of mutations.** The **pattern of replication** for major viruses is shown in **Table 20-1.** *Note:* For all ss RNA viruses (except retroviruses), a homologous replicative intermediate is required.

D. **Viral assembly.** Ultimately, all viral proteins are made and the virus is assembled.

E. **Viral release.** Virus is **released by lysis** of the cell (naked viruses) or by **budding** (enveloped viruses, as shown in **Figure 20-5**). Enveloped viruses with **fusion proteins** may enter an adjoining cell by fusion of the two cell membranes, creating giant cell syncytia and avoiding the extracellular environment (and the immune system) entirely.

IV. VIRAL DISEASE PATTERNS. Generalized **patterns of viral disease** are shown in **Figure 20-6.**

A. **Acute infections.** Because they kill the cells in the release process, **naked viruses** generally just produce **acute** infections. Some enveloped viruses also cause acute infections. Some viruses (not shown in Fig. 20-6) are **acute infections with late sequelae.** For example, with measles virus, subacute sclerosing panencephalitis may occur many years after the initial acute infection.

B. **Chronic infections.** These productive infections (with continued viral release generally lasting >6 months) **are most commonly enveloped viruses** such as hepatitis B.

C. **Latent infections.** Latent infections (with viral nucleic acid **present** in a cell **but not actively producing virus** except under certain conditions) occur with some viruses, like herpes simplex. (*Note:* HIV is *not* considered to be a latent virus. After active early viral replication, the cells continue to produce a low level of virus unless effectively treated with antiviral drugs.)

V. CHARACTERISTICS OF HEPATITIS VIRUS AND DISEASE. All five hepatitis viruses and their diseases are shown in **Table 20-2.**

A. All hepatitis viruses are **either RNA viruses** (hepatitis A, C, D, and E) **or a DNA virus replicating through an RNA intermediate** (hepatitis B.)

Steps in Generalized Viral Infection

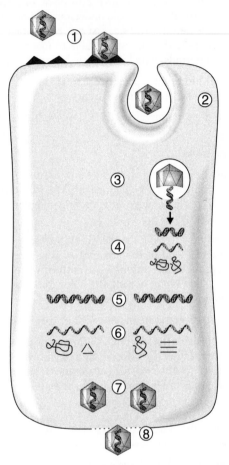

1. Attachment - specific viral outer proteins (or glycoproteins on envelope viruses) bind to chemical groups on cell membrane

2. Virus uptake by pinocytosis (as shown) or by fusion of the viral envelope with the cytoplasmic membrane

3. Uncoating (nucleic acid released)

4. Early mRNA and protein (to shut off host synthesis and make any needed enzymes)

5. Duplication of nucleic acid

6. Late mRNA and protein

7. Assembly and intracellular virus accumulation

8. Release by lysis or by budding out of cell membrane (if enveloped)

Stages 2-6 Eclipse Phase–no internal or external virus
Stages 2-7 Latent Phase–no external virus

Figure 20-2.   Viral replication overview of a generalized infection. The **eclipse period** is the time **from up-take** of the virus **to just before the assembly of the first intracellular virus (steps 2–6).** The **latent period** is the time from the **initial infection to** just prior to the **first release of the extracellular virus (steps 2–7).**

The One-Step Viral Growth Curve

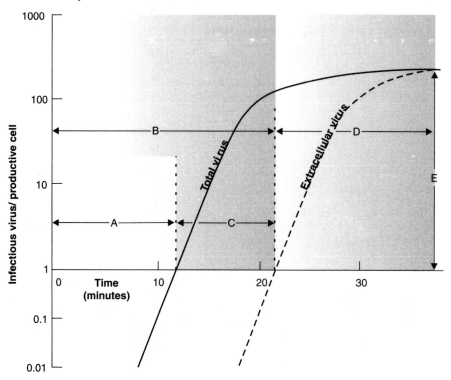

Figure 20-3.   The one-step growth curve. Cells were infected; the remaining free virus was removed. Only complete, assembled virus was detected. At each time point two samples were taken: (1) Supernatant (no cells) was assayed for free extracellular virus. (2) The entire sample (media and cells) was lysed and assayed for total virus, which included intra- and extracellular virus. **A = Eclipse period. B = Latent period. C = Intracellular accumulation period. D = Rise period** (time it takes to release all the virus). **E = Viral yield** (number of virus per cell).

Production of Viral mRNA

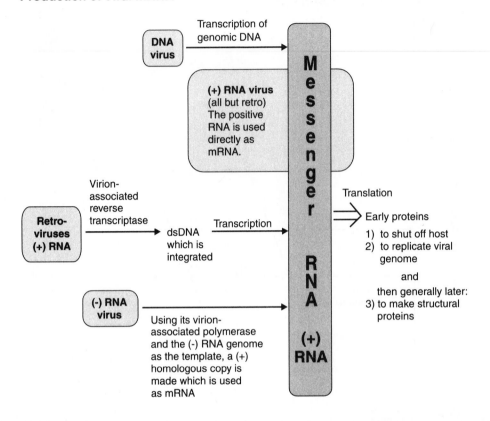

Figure 20-4. Scheme by which various viral groups make their early viral mRNA.

Table 20-1
Synthesis of Viral Nucleic Acid

Genome	Replication	New Genomes (same as original)
dsDNA	DNA separates, with each half serving as the template to produce new double strands (ds).	dsDNA
+ RNA (except retroviruses)	Makes a (−) homologous strand (using its RNA-dependent RNA polymerase, which it has made as on one of its early proteins). Then the (−) homolog serves as template to make more (+) RNA.	(+)RNA
Retroviruses (+RNA)	Using virion-associated reverse transcriptase, a dsDNA is made and integrated into the host cell's chromosome. Intact RNA transcripts serve as new genomes.	(+)RNA (retroviral)
(−)RNA	Using the virion-associated, RNA-dependent, (−) RNA polymerase, a (+) replicative intermediate is made. The (+) homolog is used to make more (−) RNA.	(−)RNA

Viral Encapsulation

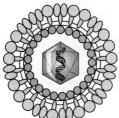

1. Virus synthesizes surface glycoproteins, which are inserted into the cell membrane of the infected cell. These glycoproteins are required for the virus to infect cells. In these viruses, the underlying icosahedron does not have viral proteins to adhere to cells.

2. Viral nucleocapsid (and matrix proteins if the virus has any) builds up by membrane.

3. Nucleocapsid buds out, taking a piece of the host cell membrane, but not lysing the cell. This is why some enveloped viruses are able to cause persistent infections.

4. Mature virion is released.

Figure 20-5.   Viral encapsulation. All surface glycoproteins added to the membrane (shaded *dark* in the figure) are viral coded.

Patterns of Viral Disease

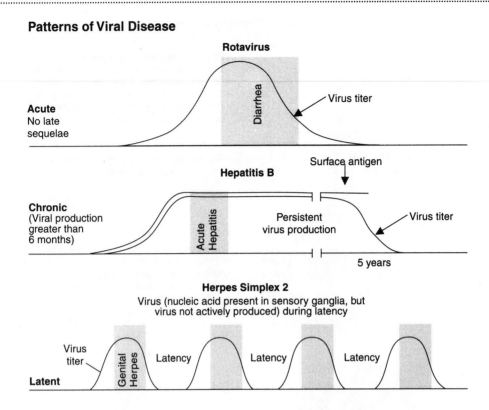

Figure 20-6.   Patterns of basic viral disease. The *gray boxes* show the disease state, and the *lines* show the viral titers.

Table 20-2
Comparison of Hepatitis Viruses

Name	Viral Characteristics	Distinguishing Features
Hepatitis A	Picornavirus: positive ss RNA Naked icosahedral	"Infectious" hepatitis Fecal-oral, often food-borne Onset generally abrupt, disease mild; 0.5% mortality No chronic infections; no association with cancer
Hepatitis E	Calicivirus: positive ss RNA Naked icosahedral	"Enteric" hepatitis Fecal-oral, often food-borne Normal people: onset abrupt, disease mild; 1–2% mortality Pregnant patient: severe; 20% mortality No chronic infections; no association with cancer
Hepatitis B	Hepadnavirus: enveloped, partially ds Circular DNA Replicates through an RNA intermediate	"Serum" hepatitis Parenteral or sexual transmission Insidious onset common; disease may be severe, with 1%–2% mortality Associated with primary hepatocellular carcinoma, cirrhosis
Hepatitis C	Flavivirus: enveloped positive ss RNA virus	"Post-transfusion" hepatitis Parenteral or sexual transmission Acute disease usually subclinical, but high rate of chronicity with 1%–2% mortality Associated with primary hepatocellular carcinoma, cirrhosis
Hepatitis D	Defective enveloped RNA virus Requires hepatitis B as helper virus to replicate	"Delta" hepatitis Co-infection (both acquired at same time) occasionally severe Superinfection (patient already infected with B then acquires B and D), high mortality: cirrhosis, fulminant hepatitis

B. The **fecally–orally transmitted** hepatitis viruses (A and E) are both **naked** and are resistant to stomach acid. Neither A nor E sets up chronic infections.

C. The **enveloped hepatitis** viruses are all **blood-borne,** may be transmitted sexually, and all have the **potential to become chronic.** Chronic hepatitis increases the risk of primary hepatocellular carcinoma.

D. Hepatitis D is a **defective RNA virus** that **requires hepatitis B to replicate. Co-infections** (B and D acquired together) **are serious. Superinfections** (i.e., when a person already has hepatitis B and then acquires hepatitis B again with D) are even **more likely to be fatal.**

E. **Acute signs of hepatitis** generally include fever, malaise, headache, dark urine, vomiting, and jaundice.

21

DNA Viruses

Parvoviruses, Papovaviruses, Adenoviruses, Hepadnaviruses, Herpesviruses, Poxviruses

I. HIGH-YIELD CONCEPTS

A. All DNA viruses except the parvoviruses are **double-stranded (ds).**

B. All except the poxviruses **duplicate** their DNA **in the nucleus** and are **icosahedral.**

C. Naked DNA viruses are parvoviruses, adenoviruses, and papovaviruses.

D. Table 21-1 provides more details about both **naked and enveloped** DNA viruses.

II. REPLICATION

A. DNA viruses (except hepatitis B virus) duplicate their DNA by using it as a template to make more DNA.

B. **Hepatitis B** is an enveloped ds DNA virus that makes an **RNA intermediate.** [🔟 Is it peer pressure from all the other hepatitis viruses (all RNA viruses replicating through RNA intermediates) that makes them all replicate through an RNA intermediate?] A polymerase, which is very similar to the retroviral reverse transcriptase, makes the new DNA from the RNA intermediate.

III. PARVOVIRUS B19

A. B19 is a naked **single-stranded (ss) DNA** virus that causes fifth disease.

B. **Fifth disease (erythema infectiosum,** a.k.a. **slapped cheek fever)** most often infects adolescents, causing **mild fever** and a recurring **slapped cheek appearance with lacy rash** on arms and then body. It may cause chronic anemia in immunocompromised patients and aplastic crises in sickle cell patients. It can also cause hydrops fetalis.

IV. PAPOVAVIRUSES. Papovaviruses are **naked ds circular** DNA viruses that include two groups: the **papilloma (wart) viruses** and the **polyomaviruses.** (🔟 Warts are circular and you have to get "naked" to get the sexually transmitted human papilloma virus (HPV). Also, the end result of some HPV infections is a positive <u>Pap</u> test.)

A. **Human papillomaviruses** cause warts. They are transmitted by direct contact.

1. **Plantar warts** are caused by **HPV 1 and 4,** both benign.

2. HPV 6 and 11 are the most common cause of **anogenital warts (condylomata acuminata,** which are sexually transmitted) and laryngeal warts (generally seen in

Table 21-1
DNA Viruses*

Virus Family	DNA type	Virion-associated Polymerase?	Envelope?	Shape	DNA replicates in:	Major Viruses
Parvo-virus	ssDNA	No	Naked	Icosahedral	Nucleus	B-19
Papova-virus	dsDNA circular	No	Naked	Icosahedral	Nucleus	Papilloma Polyoma
Adeno-virus	dsDNA linear	No	Naked	Icosahedral	Nucleus	Adenoviruses
Hepadna-virus	dsDNA circular (part ds)	Yes**	Enveloped	Icosahedral	Nucleus	Hepatitis B
Herpes virus	dsDNA linear	No	Enveloped (nuclear)	Icosahedral	Nucleus	HSV Varicella-Zoster Epstein-Barr Cytomegalovirus
Poxvirus	dsDNA linear	Yes***	Enveloped (makes own)	Brick-shaped complex	Cytoplasm	Variola Vaccinia Molluscum contagiosum

* Mnemonic: Poor Poppie Adds Hop to Her Pox.

** Hepadnavirus replicates through an RNA intermediate which is used as the template to make more DNA. Therefore it carries its own DNA polymerase, which has RNA-dependent DNA polymerase activity.

*** A transcriptase, so that all the enzymes used for making and transcribing DNA are out in the cytoplasm where poxviruses replicate.

very young children and sometimes acquired at birth). They are problematic, **regrowing after removal, but benign.**

3. Cervical intraepithelial carcinoma is most commonly associated with **HPV 16 and 18.** The **early proteins of these oncogenic HPVs, E6 and E7, inactivate tumor suppressor functions of p53 and p110-Rb, respectively.**

B. Polyomaviruses BK and JC are common but cause disease only in compromised patients. **BK virus** causes **kidney disease** and is often associated with kidney transplantation. **JC virus** is associated with **progressive multifocal leukoencephalopathy.**

V. ADENOVIRUSES

A. Adenoviruses are **naked icosahedral ds DNA viruses with fibers** projecting from the penton subunits of the capsid. Adenoviruses have serotype numbers.

B. Adenoviruses cause a variety of **childhood and adult diseases,** such as:

   1. **Pharygoconjunctivitis and keratoconjunctivitis.** Unlike bacterial pink eye, **adenoviral pink eye** is **not purulent;** the conjunctivae are inflamed with a watery exudate.

   2. **Acute respiratory diseases.** The most serious is **interstitial pneumonitis in immunocompromised patients.** The military has had to combat major problems with adenoviral respiratory disease in young recruits; one unique, **new and effective vaccine** consists of the virulent respiratory strains of adenovirus administered orally in enteric-coated capsules.

   3. Adenoviruses 40 and 41 cause **gastroenteritis.**

VI. HEPADNAVIRUS

A. **Hepatitis B virus is an enveloped, partially ds DNA virus.** Because it replicates through an RNA intermediate, it carries **in the mature virus particle (virion) a DNA polymerase** with reverse transcriptase and DNA-dependent DNA polymerase activity. The genomic DNA is first transcribed into an RNA intermediate. Then the RNA is copied (using the reverse transcriptase) into the new genomic partially stranded DNA.

B. **Transmission.** Hepatitis B is parenterally or sexually transmitted.

C. **Disease** may be acute or chronic. (**Chronic disease** is indicated by **presence of $HB_sAg > 6$ months.**) The **correlation of various antigens and antibodies with the presence of virus** and symptomology is shown in **Figure 21-1.** *Note:* Patients with chronic infections are, on average, infectious for about 5 years and are unable to suppress the production of HB_sAg.

D. **Diagnosis** is made by serology, testing for the presence of IgM to HB_cAg, anti-HB_sAg, and HB_sAg. HB_eAg's presence correlates well to the presence of virus. The presence of **anti-HB_eAg indicates a lower risk of transmission** of the virus.

VII. HERPESVIRUSES. This family of large, enveloped, icosahedral, ds DNA viruses includes the herpes simplex viruses (HSV), varicella-zoster virus (VZV), Epstein-Barr virus (EBV), and cytomegalovirus (CMV). Viruses of the **herpes** family are the **only viruses assembled in the nucleus** of the infected cell and the **only ones whose envelope is from host cell nuclear membrane modified by viral glycoproteins.** Herpesviruses may become latent; HSV and VZV both become latent in neurons.

A. **Herpes simplex viruses (HSVs).** HSVs may cause either acute or latent infections.

   1. **Latent infections.** The HSV **DNA** is present **in nerve ganglia, and alpha (immediate early) proteins are expressed,** but the **beta viral proteins** such as the **HSV thymidine kinase** and **DNA polymerase** (required for new DNA synthesis and for virus production) are not made. Thus, anti-HSV drugs like acyclovir, which inhibit the DNA polymerase, do not wipe out latent infections.

   2. **Lesions.** Both HSV-1 and HSV-2 are noted for **initially vesicular cutaneous lesions.** A gross generalization is that **HSV-1 is usually above the waist and HSV-2, below.** HSV-1 is most noted for causing gingivostomatitis, keratoconjunctivitis, and meningitis. HSV-2 is noted for genital herpes or neonatal infections.

   3. **HSV-1.** Infections are often asymptomatic initially or manifest as **gingivostomatitis** (fever with painful oral vesicles or ulcers), usually in 3- to 5-year-olds. The virus may become latent in the trigeminal nerve ganglia and recur periodically as

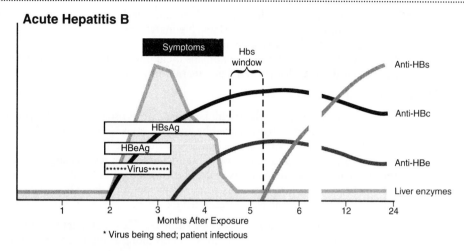

Acute Hepatitis B

Symptoms

Hbs
window

Anti-HBs

Anti-HBc

HBsAg

HBeAg

Anti-HBe

******Virus******

Liver enzymes

1   2   3   4   5   6   12   24

Months After Exposure

* Virus being shed; patient infectious

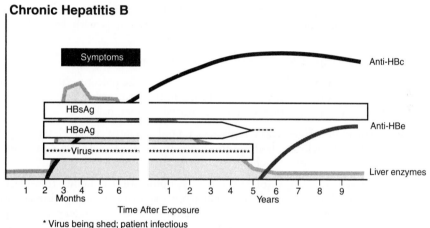

Chronic Hepatitis B

Symptoms

Anti-HBc

HBsAg

HBeAg

Anti-HBe

*******Virus***************   *****************************

Liver enzymes

1 2 3 4 5 6   1   2   3   4   5   6   7   8   9

Months   Years

Time After Exposure

* Virus being shed; patient infectious

Figure 21-1.   A comparison of virus production, antigens, antibodies, and symptoms of acute and chronic hepatitis B virus infections. These studies were important to allow serological diagnosis. Note that the hepatitis B "e" antigen correlates with presence of virus (infectivity) and that as soon as the virus disappears, the antibody to "e" rises. Also note that there is a time period when neither the "s" antigen nor the "s" antibody is detected; the antibody to "c" is used so as not to miss the diagnosis of hepatitis B virus.

cold sores or **fever blisters.** Herpes may infect a finger or nail area causing **herpetic whitlow. Herpetic ulcers of the cornea or conjunctivae** may cause blindness. **HSV-1 is the most common cause of sporadic encephalitis;** CSF may be normal, but the finding in CSF of slightly elevated lymphocytes and protein and red cells is suggestive. PCR on CSF is the diagnostic method of choice. Rapid diagnosis and administration of acyclovir have reduced mortality.

4. HSV-2. It is **sexually transmitted,** may be asymptomatic (both primary and recurrent), **localizes in sacral nerve ganglia,** and may cause painful primary outbreaks and exacerbations with **tingling prior to new outbreaks of vesicular lesions,** which ulcerate; regional lymphadenopathy occurs. Because of the risk of serious neonatal disease, delivery by C-section is indicated in the presence of active cervical, vaginal, or labial lesions. **Neonatal herpes** may be:

a. **Localized to skin, eyes, or mouth**

b. **Generalized,** involving many organs including the lungs, liver, and CNS

c. **Localized to CNS** without other manifestations

B. **Varicella-zoster virus (VZV)**

1. **Primary infection: varicella or chickenpox.** This is usually a **mild febrile disease** (in normal children), characterized by asynchronous appearance of discrete, erythematous papular lesions on mucocutaneous surfaces. The lesions vesiculate, develop into pustules, and crust over while new crops of lesions appear, producing the characteristic **asynchronous rash.** The virus becomes latent. Incubation time is 13 to 17 days. Children are considered contagious for 6 days after all lesions have dried. The **VZV vaccine** is an **attenuated** ("live" but modified) strain of the virus.

2. **Secondary infection: herpes zoster or shingles.** This is characterized by the appearance of clusters of vesicular lesions, usually along a single sensory dermatome.

3. **Immunocompromised patients.** Both chickenpox and shingles are much more severe in immunocompromised patients. Treatment is with varicella zoster immunoglobulin (VZIG) and oral acyclovir.

C. **Cytomegalovirus (CMV).** CMV is **extremely common.**

1. **Transmission.** CMV may be transferred across the placenta (in either primary or reactivated infection), acquired during birth or through mother's milk, or transferred by direct contact with others, sexual contact, or blood.

2. **Replication.** When CMV replicates, it produces large cells with typical purple intranuclear inclusion bodies surrounded by a halo ("owl's eye") and smaller basophilic cytoplasmic inclusions.

3. **Disease.** Most CMV infections are **asymptomatic** (including transplacental infections), but they may be mononucleosis-like in adults. CMV **clinical disease** includes **retinitis and interstitial pneumonitis in immunocompromised patients;** infections in immunocompromised people are severe. In neonates infected very early, **cytomegalic inclusion disease** may develop (hepatosplenomegaly with thrombocytopenic purpura, pneumonitis, and CNS calcifications and microcephaly).

D. **Epstein-Barr virus (EBV)**

1. EBV is also a Herpesviridae (herpes family), which infects by **binding to CD21** molecules on human **B lymphocytes.** Several antigens have been useful, including the EB nuclear antigens (EBNA), early antigens (EA), and viral capsid antigen (VCA).

2. In the U.S., **EB infectious mononucleosis (IM)** is most commonly found in 15- to 25-year-olds. It presents as severe **fatigue, pharyngitis/tonsillitis** similar to strep throat, **postcervical lymphadenopathy, hepatomegaly** (with elevated alkaline phosphatase), and **splenomegaly.** There is a dramatic mononucleosis, presence of reactive Downey type II cells (thymus derived), and the formation of **heterophile antibodies** (unique to EBV infections), which react with animal red blood cell antigens (rather than the virus). Heterophile antibody tests (e.g., Monospot) or tests for specific EBV antibodies to EA or VCA are available.

VIII. POXVIRUSES. Poxviruses are very **large** and unusual ds DNA viruses, often described as having a **brick-shaped complex** appearance. Poxviruses make all nucleic acids in the cytoplasm. They require a **virion-associated transcriptase** in order to make the various viral enzymes to synthesize all their nucleic acids. (All cellular polymerases, ligases, and so on are located in the nucleus, so they cannot be used.) The poxviruses also direct the synthesis of their own envelopes, rather than just modifying human cell membranes. Infection with poxviruses produces **cytoplasmic inclusion bodies.**

A. **Variola** was the virus that caused smallpox. It has been extinct in the wild since 1977. (● You should never see the typical intracytoplasmic inclusion bodies, called Guarnieri bodies, since they have "guone" away.)

B. **Vaccinia virus** was the **immunogen in the vaccine** that led to the successful eradication of smallpox. Vaccinia is of uncertain origin.

C. **Molluscum contagiosum,** another poxvirus, causes benign, pincushionlike, pink tumors with nipplelike indentations. Virus-infected cells have large eosinophilic cytoplasmic inclusion bodies called **molluscum bodies.** This virus can be a problem in seriously compromised patients.

22

Positive ss RNA (+RNA) Viruses

I. HIGH-YIELD CONCEPTS

A. Definition. Positive RNA (+RNA) viruses are those viruses whose genomic RNA either serves directly as mRNA (all positive RNA viruses except the retroviruses) or has the same sequence as the mRNA (retroviruses). All +RNA viruses (again, except the retroviruses) carry the genetic code for an RNA-dependent RNA polymerase but do *not* carry the polymerase protein in the mature virion, because they can make it immediately in the host cell.

B. Characteristics

1. Naked +RNA is infectious.

2. Positive RNA viruses (except retrovirus) replicate in the cytoplasm.

3. No +RNA virus is segmented.

4. The retroviruses are diploid (two copies of the chromosome).

5. All RNA viruses are enveloped except the smallest, the caliciviruses and picornaviruses.

C. Viral families. See **Table 22-1.**

II. PICORNAVIRIDAE. Picornaviruses are a large group of **very small, naked icosahedral, positive ss RNA viruses,** all of which replicate through a negative strand intermediate. Picornaviruses have very tightly fitting capsid protein subunits (capsomers) which are involved in cell binding and are **hard to inactivate with disinfectants or organic solvents.** (None of the required cell-binding proteins is held in place by lipid, as occurs in the enveloped viruses.) Picornaviruses are divided into the Enterovirus genus (poliovirus, coxsackievirus, echovirus, enteroviruses 68–71, and hepatitis A, all of which survive stomach acid) and the rhinoviruses, which are acid-labile. (● A mnemonic for the picornaviruses is **PEECoRnA:** <u>P</u>olio, <u>E</u>ntero, <u>E</u>cho, <u>Co</u>xsackie, <u>R</u>hi<u>n</u>o, and hepatitis <u>A</u>.)

A. Poliovirus

1. Transmission. Poliovirus is transmitted by the **fecal-oral route.**

2. Serotypes. There are **three stable** polioviruses (1, 2, and 3) which may be eradicated through the use of the oral **(attenuated) Sabin** or the <u>k</u>illed **(Sal<u>k</u>)** vaccines.

3. Disease. The virus infects oral and GI epithelium; 90% to 95% of the infections are asymptomatic. When it infects the anterior horn cells of the spinal cord (1/250 infections), poliovirus may cause a paralytic disease involving the cranial and respiratory nerves. Because of cases of vaccine-associated paralytic poliomyelitis (i.e.,

Table 22-1

Positive-Sense RNA Viruses

Virus family*	RNA Structure	Virion-associated Polymerase?	Envelope?	Shape	Multiplies in	Major Viruses
Picorna-virus	ss(+)RNA Linear nonsegmented	No polymerase	Naked	Icosahedral	Cytoplasm	Polio, Echo, Entero, Rhino, Coxsackievirus, Hepatitis A
Calici-virus	ss(+)RNA Linear nonsegmented	No polymerase	Naked	Icosahedral		Norwalk agent Hepatitis E
Flavi-virus	ss(+)RNA Linear nonsegmented	No polymerase	Enveloped	Icosahedral	Cytoplasm	Yellow fever, Dengue St. Louis encephalitis Hepatitis C
Toga-virus	ss(+)RNA Linear nonsegmented	No polymerase	Enveloped	Icosahedral	Cytoplasm	Rubella, W. & E. equine encephalitis, Venezuelan encephalitis
Corona-virus	ss(+)RNA Linear nonsegmented	No polymerase	Enveloped	Helical	Cytoplasm	Coronaviruses
Retro-virus	Diploid ss(+)RNA Linear nonsegmented	RNA-dep. DNA polymerase	Enveloped	Icosahedral or truncated conical	Nucleus	HIV Human T cell lympho-trophic virus Sarcoma

*Mnemonic: **Pico Calls Flavio To Come Right Away.**

caused by the vaccine strain), the U.S. now uses the killed vaccine for at least the first two doses. Culture with serology is used to determine whether cases are vaccine-associated.

B. **Other enteroviruses (Coxsackie A and B, enteroviruses 68–71, and echoviruses)** are common and significant causative agents of:

1. **Upper respiratory infections (URIs)** such as colds, herpangina, and stomatitis. Herpangina is characterized by gray-white papulovesicles on anterior tonsillar pillars and tonsils, soft palate, and uvula.

2. **Rashes and vesicles,** such as hand-foot-and-mouth disease, a vesicular disease

3. **CNS infections**—most often meningitis, less commonly encephalitis. Viral meningitis (generally benign) presents with fever, headache, stiff neck, and malaise. CSF cell counts are 0 to 500 cells/mm^3 (initially PMNs predominate, then lymphocytes); glucose is generally near normal and protein is normal or only slightly elevated.

4. **Gastrointestinal disorders**

5. **Hemorrhagic conjunctivitis**

6. **Myopericarditis** (caused primarily by Coxsackie B and characterized by chest pains, fever, fatigue, and arrhythmias)

C. **Hepatitis A** is a Picornavirus. (For a review of hepatitis viruses, see Table 20-2.)

D. **Rhinoviruses** are the major causative agents of the common cold. They peak in the summer and early fall.

III. CALICIVIRIDAE. Caliciviruses are **naked icosahedral positive ss RNA viruses** slightly larger than the picornaviruses. These viruses are the causative agents in the diseases described below.

A. **Norwalk gastroenteritis** is a **noninflammatory diarrhea** found in older children and adults. It often is spread at **potluck meals** or by **contaminated shellfish** but may be water-borne in developing countries. There is generally a 1- to 2-day incubation and 1 day of illness, with vomiting, diarrhea, and a low-grade fever.

B. **Hepatitis E** (see Table 20-2) has **a high fatality rate in pregnant women.**

IV. FLAVIVIRIDAE are **enveloped, icosahedral positive ss RNA viruses.** Flaviviruses are the causative agents in the diseases described below.

A. **Hepatitis C.** Often initially asymptomatic, hepatitis C has a **high rate of chronicity** (see Table 20-2). **Diagnosis** is by screening enzyme immunoassay with a recombinant immunoblot (like HIV diagnosis), as well as PCR for RNA. **Treatment** is with interferon alpha.

B. **Yellow fever.** The yellow fever virus (tropical South America and Africa) is spread by **mosquitoes** (*a*rthropod-*bo*rne virus = arbovirus). It causes febrile disease of varying severity, which often includes hepatitis and may progress to hemorrhagic fever. The **vaccine** is attenuated.

C. **Dengue.** The dengue virus is another arbovirus belonging to the Flaviviridae. Dengue (breakbone disease) is spread by **Aedes mosquitoes** in the tropics. Clinically it has a rapid onset with **fever, severe myalgias, arthralgias, headache, and rash.** There are four serotypes. **Dengue hemorrhagic shock syndrome** is a serious complication often seen in young children with previous antibodies and now infected with a second dengue fever serotype.

D. St. Louis encephalitis. The **mosquito-spread** encephalitis virus is endemic in Canada, the U.S., the Caribbean, and South America. The disease is **most severe in the elderly.**

V. TOGAVIRIDAE. Togaviruses are **enveloped, icosahedral positive ss RNA viruses.**

A. Alphaviruses include the **Western, Eastern, and Venezuelan equine encephalitis (EE) viruses.** Horses are dead-end hosts; **wild birds** are the normal hosts. **Mosquitoes** transfer the disease to humans.

B. Rubella virus causes **German measles,** which is characterized by a discrete red maculopapular rash, lymphadenopathy, and mild fever. The virus can cross the placenta and cause **serious birth defects** such as cataracts and retinopathy, patent ductus arteriosus, and sensorineural deafness.

VI. CORONAVIRIDAE. Coronaviruses are **larger, enveloped, helical, positive ss RNA viruses** which are divided into **antigenic groups.** The envelope has prominent surface glycoproteins (hemagglutinins); the virus resembles a crown (hence "corona"). Coronaviruses are the second most common causative agents of the common cold, appearing mainly in winter and spring.

VII. RETROVIRIDAE. Retroviruses are **diploid, enveloped positive ss RNA viruses. Mature virions carry the reverse transcriptase and integrase proteins,** as well as those for the nucleocapsid/capsid, within the envelope. **Human immunodeficiency virus (HIV),** currently the medically most important retrovirus, is discussed below.

A. Genes[1] and gene products of importance in HIV infection

1. The *gag* gene (group specific antigens) codes for the structural proteins **p24 (capsid), p7 and p9 (nucleocapsid proteins), and p17 (matrix protein,** which is membrane stabilizing).

2. The *env* gene codes for gp120 **(binds CD4)** and gp41 **(transmembrane protein).**

3. The *pol* gene codes for the **reverse transcriptase** and the **integrase.**

4. The *pro* gene codes for the **protease,** which clips large protein precursors into the functional proteins (e.g., gp160 *env* gene product is cleaved by the protease into the functional gp120 and gp41).

5. **Long terminal repeats** (LTRs) are critical to integration and regulate transcription (via active enhancer promoter regions).

6. **Additional regulatory genes** are mainly positive regulators, except *nef.*

B. Events of HIV infection in an untreated person

1. **HIV gp120 binds to CD4 molecules.** Membrane fusion involving gp41 allows **nucleocapsid entry** followed by release of the genomic RNA. The **reverse transcriptase makes the dsDNA "copy,"** which migrates into the cell nucleus. The **integrase integrates the viral DNA** into the human chromosome.

2. Following transcription and production of early proteins, **HIV proteins regulate transcription, RNA cleavage and transport of RNA** to the ribosomes, and **protein cleavage,** all of which play roles in controlling viral production. The cleaved mRNAs are transported to the cytoplasm along with the intact genomic RNAs. After the proteins are made, **gp120 and gp41 are inserted into the host cyto-**

---

[1]Gene abbreviations are italicized, as is standard.

plasmic membrane. The **virus is assembled; it matures through the membrane** to pick up the envelope.

3. Clinically, there is an **initial acute mononucleosis-like disease** with high titers of virus, followed by a relatively asymptomatic period with low blood titers once the immune system is primed. **Infections with other organisms** that activate infected T-cells (e.g., hepatitis B or tuberculosis) **increase production of HIV.** When CD4+ cell counts (and antibodies to HIV) decline, viral production goes up.

C. **Opportunistic infections.** Most serious infections become major problems **at a CD4 level below 200 mm³.** Major infective organisms are listed below. Routine **prophylaxis** is used to prevent *Pneumocystis*, *M. avium-intracellulare*, and *Toxoplasma* infections.

1. **Fungal infections** include *Candida* (oral thrush → gastritis → septicemia), cryptococcal meningitis (encapsulated yeast in CSF), *Histoplasma* or *Coccidioides* (depending on exposure, sometimes years earlier), and *Pneumocystis* infections.

2. **Bacterial infections** include disseminating pulmonary infections with **Mycobacterium tuberculosis** and **M. avium-intracellulare,** as well as gastroenteritis caused by *Salmonella*, *Shigella*, and *Campylobacter*.

3. **Viral infections** include **HSV1 and HSV2 infections,** and **CMV chorioretinitis and pneumonia.**

4. **Protozoan infections** with **Cryptosporidium, Giardia, Toxoplasma,** and **Entamoeba** are common.

23

Negative ss RNA (−RNA) Viruses

I. HIGH-YIELD CONCEPTS

   A. Negative-sense RNA (−RNA) is the homolog of mRNA.

   B. All negative ss RNA viruses carry a virion-associated, RNA-dependent RNA polymerase which directs production of the positive RNA homolog used both as mRNA and as a template to make more negative copies for progeny virus.

   C. Naked −RNA (without the RNA-dependent RNA polymerase protein) is not infectious. Humans do not have RNA-dependent RNA polymerase.

   D. All −RNA viruses are helical and enveloped. None is naked; none is icosahedral.

   E. Three families of negative ss RNA viruses are segmented: the Orthomyxoviridae, the Bunyaviridae, and the Arenaviridae. The double-stranded (ds) RNA viruses (Reoviridae) are also segmented. ⊛ ROBA (like robots, made of pieces): Reoviridae, Orthomyxoviridae, Bunyaviridae, Arenaviridae. The −RNA viral families are shown in Table 23-1.

II. REPLICATION

   A. Viral surface groups held by the envelope determine how these viruses enter the host cells. Viruses with **fusion (F) proteins** fuse their viral envelope with host cell membrane to enter cells. The remaining enveloped viruses enter by a pinocytotic process triggered by the virus envelope glycoproteins (such as hemagglutinins) binding to host cell receptors.

   B. Envelope glycoproteins also identify viruses as hemagglutinating or nonhemagglutinating. In terms of host antibody response, if the **hemagglutinin (H)** and **neuraminidase (N)** are separate, each stimulates a separate antibody. [*Note:* This is important in vaccine or protection questions (e.g., influenza A/H1N1). The presence of a number between an H and N designation should remind you that these are separate antigens.]

III. PARAMYXOVIRUSES are large, enveloped, helical, negative ss RNA viruses. They
all have a single dominant serotype, except for the parainfluenza viruses, which have four. All are transmitted via respiratory secretion, directly or by fomites.

   A. Measles virus (rubeola)

      1. Rubeola has H, F (no N), and a virion-associated polymerase.

      2. **Common presentation** is **fever, cough, coryza, conjunctivitis, Koplik's spots (gray white with red base on oral mucosa),** and an erythematous maculopapular

Table 23-1
Negative-Sense RNA Viruses

Virus*	RNA structure	Virion-associated Polymerase?	Envelope?	Shape	Multiplies in	Major Viruses
Para-myxovirus	Linear nonsegmented ss(-)RNA	Yes**	Yes	Helical spikes: HN&F glycoprotein	Cytoplasm	Measles Mumps, Respiratory syncytial Parainfluenza
Rhabdo-virus	Linear nonsegmented ss(-)RNA	Yes	Yes	Bullet-shaped helical	Cytoplasm	Rabies Vesicular stomatitis
Filovirus	Linear nonsegmented ss(-)RNA	Yes	Yes	Helical		Marburg Ebola
Ortho-myxovirus	Linear 8 segments ss(-)RNA	Yes	Yes	Helical	Cytoplasm & nucleus	Influenza
Bunyavirus	Linear 3 segments: 2 ss(-)RNA ambisense	Yes	Yes	Helical	Cytoplasm	California encephalitis (La Crosse) Hanta, Hataan
Arenavirus	Circular 2 segments: 1 ss(-) sense 1 ambisense RNA	Yes	Yes	Helical	Cytoplasm	Lymphocytic choriomeningitis Lassa fever

* Mnemonic: **Para R**abbits **F**ight **O**ver **B**unnies' **A**rea.

** In all cases RNA-dependent RNA polymerase.

rash (a result of the action of cytotoxic T cells on infected cells in the microcapillaries). The rash starts on the face and moves down, becoming quite confluent.

3. **Complications** (more common in younger children) include otitis media, bronchopneumonia with giant cells (Warthin-Finkeldey cells), and diarrhea. The more severe problems occur in malnourished children (vitamin A treatment increases survival) and in immunocompromised patients.

4. The **vaccine** is an attenuated strain.

B. **Mumps virus** has combined HN, F, and a virion-associated polymerase. Clinical disease includes **salivary gland enlargement** in most cases, **meningeal signs,** and **orchitis** (postpuberty, and rarely causing sterility). The **vaccine** is attenuated.

C. **Parainfluenza virus,** like mumps, has combined HN, F, and a virion-associated polymerase. It causes **croup** (laryngotracheobronchitis) in infants, URIs, pneumonia, and bronchiolitis. There are four serotypes, and **no vaccine.**

D. **Respiratory syncytial virus (RSV)** is an enveloped negative ss RNA virus with **only a fusion (F) protein.** RSV is the **major cause of bronchiolitis and pneumonia in infants and young children;** it causes colds with bronchitis in older children, adolescents, and adults.

IV. RHABDOVIRIDAE

A. **Rabies virus** is an **enveloped negative RNA virus** with a **helical nucleocapsid** and overall **bullet shape.**

1. **Reservoirs and transmission.** Rabies reservoirs in the U.S. are skunks (West), raccoons or foxes (East), coyotes or dogs (Texas-Mexico border), and bats (throughout the U.S.). Rabies is generally transmitted to humans by **bat contact or dog bite** (an unvaccinated dog having acquired it from a reservoir). Rodents and rabbits rarely carry rabies. Over the past 20 years, about 25% of the human rabies deaths in the U.S. resulted from animal bites (89% of cases from dog bites). From 1980 on, all strains from human deaths in the U.S. in which no bite was known were typed; more than half were found to be insectivorous bat strains.

2. **Disease prevention.** Rabies virus grows through neurons, so if the bite site is far from the CNS, **postexposure use of hyperimmune serum and the killed vaccine** may prevent disease.

3. **Negri bodies** are the eosinophilic intracytoplasmic inclusion bodies seen in tissues.

B. **Vesicular stomatitis virus** is an arbovirus (*a*rthropod-*b*orne virus) that causes foot-and-mouth disease, uncommon in humans.

V. FILOVIRIDAE. These viruses (a.k.a. "thread" viruses) are long helical, enveloped, negative ss viruses. Both **Ebola** and **Marburg** viruses are causative agents of **hemorrhagic fever,** a disease that starts with influenzalike symptoms, then vomiting and diarrhea, and often ends with severe bleeding, shock, and death.

VI. ORTHOMYXOVIRIDAE (INFLUENZA A AND B VIRUSES)

A. **Structure.** Influenza A and B viruses are **enveloped negative ss RNA segmented viruses** with **eight helical segments. Separate** viral coded **H and N** glycoproteins stud the envelope surface, playing the usual roles in cell binding and release. The hemagglutinin appears to induce the most protective antibodies.

B. **Genetic drift.** Because the RNA-dependent RNA polymerase makes errors without repairing them, the resulting minor surface antigen changes (referred to as genetic drift) mandate an annual vaccine program that updates the immune system on the newest strains of both influenza A and B viruses. (See Chapter 25, I A, for more information on genetic drift.)

C. **Genetic reassortment.** Periodically there is a dramatic antigenic change in the influenza A viruses **(called antigenic shift** or **genetic reassortment)** that leads to very large, serious outbreaks of influenza A. (*Note:* There are eight different segments of RNA or "chromosomes" in each virus.) Antigenic shift may occur when an individual is co-infected with an avian or animal A strain *and* a human A strain, and the progeny virus is assembled with some "chromosomes" of both strains. This results in the production of a dramatically new strain leading to a pandemic.

VII. **BUNYAVIRIDAE.** Bunyaviruses are **segmented, enveloped helical ss RNA viruses with two chromosomes of negative ss stranded RNA** and **one ambisense (±) chromosome.** (Some regions of ambisense RNA function like negative RNA and others like positive RNA.)

A. **California encephalitis virus** (spread by *Aedes* **spp. mosquitoes)** causes subclinical infections or occasionally **nonfatal encephalitis in school-aged children in North America in the summer and fall.** Small mammals are the reservoir hosts.

B. **Hantavirus (Sin Nombre Hantavirus)** causes an infection with an influenzalike presentation leading to acute respiratory failure (hantavirus pulmonary syndrome). It is transmitted in deer mice feces and urine.

VIII. **ARENAVIRIDAE.** Arenaviruses are **enveloped RNA viruses** with **two helical segments: one with negative RNA and one with ambisense RNA.**

A. **Lymphocytic choriomeningitis** (LCM) **virus** causes an influenzalike febrile disease with meningitis. Unlike most viral meningitis, LCM **may be fatal.**

B. Other arenaviruses cause **Lassa fever** and the South American hemorrhagic fevers (Argentinian and Bolivian). These febrile diseases are complicated by hemorrhage.

24

Double-Stranded (ds) RNA Viruses: Reoviridae

I. MAJOR CONCEPTS. Viruses of the **family Reoviridae** are **naked** and have both **double-stranded (ds) RNA** and **double-shelled icosahedral capsids.** There are 10 to 12 segments (chromosomes) of ds RNA, depending on the virus. There are three viruses of importance to humans: Rotavirus, Orbivirus, and Reovirus.

II. ROTAVIRUS. Rotaviruses are the major cause of infantile diarrhea worldwide. They produce a noninflammatory, prolonged diarrhea in babies younger than 2 years of age.

III. ORBIVIRUS. The **Colorado tick fever virus,** an Orbivirus species transmitted by *Dermacentor andersoni,* is one causative agent of viral encephalitis.

IV. REOVIRUS. Exposure to the reoviruses (sometimes called the **orthoreoviruses**) without overt disease appears to be common in humans. They may also cause a febrile disease.

25

Viral Genetics

I. MUTATION: GENETIC DRIFT AND DEFECTIVE INTERFERING PARTICLES.
Mutations are caused by genetic errors. Mutations can help viruses evade the immune system; they can also limit the duration of a viral infection. Most **viral-coded polymerases do not recognize and fix errors.** As a result, mutation rates are higher in viruses that make their own polymerases than in viruses that use human host cell polymerases. Viruses that make their own polymerases include all the RNA viruses, poxviruses, HSV, VZV, and adenoviruses. A **point mutation** is one type of genetic error. Other errors include larger deletions or additions made when the polymerases "fall off" the template and reattach at a different site on the template; this leads to **shorter or longer defective pieces of nucleic acid.** Medically important genetic errors include:

A. Genetic drift. Point mutations lead to **minor changes in antigenicity called antigenic drift.**

    1. Influenza viruses. Antigenic drift in the influenza virus hemagglutinins and neuraminidases necessitates new influenza vaccines every year.

    2. Human immunodeficiency virus (HIV). The antigenic drift in HIV's **gp120** (the major surface antigen) leads to multiple variants within one person dying of AIDS. Antigenic drift helps HIV evade the immune system and has slowed vaccine development.

B. Defective interfering particles. Virus production continues as long as there is one functional copy of every viral gene in the host cell. As replication proceeds, more defective nucleic acids are produced. Polymerases bind to both the normal *and* the defective nucleic acid pieces. The shorter defective nucleic acids replicate faster, leading to increased production of viral particles with defective nucleic acid, known as **defective interfering (DI) particles.** As infection progresses, fewer normal virions and more DI particles are produced, helping to limit the viral infection.

II. VIRAL COMPLEMENTATION. Viral complementation (co-infection of one cell with two viral genomes leading to virus production) is a genetic laboratory technique and a real-life phenomenon. Possible types include the following:

A. Co-infection with both DI particles and normal virus. This is described above in I B. As viral production proceeds, fewer normal virus and more DI particles are produced until there is no longer a functional copy of each gene in the cell.

B. Co-infection with two mutant (and no normal) strains of the same virus

    1. A continuation of virus production indicates that each mutant was defective in a *different* gene, so there was one functional copy of each gene in the cell to allow production of all proteins. (All of the virions will still have mutant nucleic acid unless recombination occurs.)

2. Lack of viral production (complementation) indicates each of the two strains was defective in the *same* gene.

C. Co-infection with defective virus and helper virus. Hepatitis D, a defective RNA virus, can only replicate in a cell co-infected with its **"helper" virus hepatitis B** (a DNA virus). Hepatitis B replication provides the surface protein that hepatitis D needs for infectivity.

III. GENE REASSORTMENT (GENETIC SHIFT) occurs with **segmented RNA viruses.** A cell infected with two different strains of a segmented virus may produce an **antigenically new virus** by incorporating RNA segments from **each parental strain.** This is best exemplified by the influenza A viruses. There are many avian and other animal strains that may co-infect with a human influenza strain to create dramatically different strains to which no one has partial immunity. This leads to worldwide outbreaks of very severe disease (pandemics), such as the influenza epidemic in 1918.

IV. LATENCY. Latent viruses exist as **stable nucleic acid** in the host cell, either **free in a plasmidlike state or integrated into the host cell genome (provirus).** Continued production of repressor proteins prevents the replication of virus.

A. Lysogenic conversion. Latency of bacteriophage in bacterial cells is called **lysogeny** (see Chapter 5). Lysogenic conversion occurs when, in addition to the repressor protein, other phage genes are expressed, **making the bacterium virulent.** Medically important examples are modification of *Salmonella* <u>O</u> antigens and production of <u>b</u>otulinum toxin, the <u>e</u>rythrogenic toxins of *Streptococcus pyogenes* (SPE-A, B, or C), and <u>d</u>iphtheria toxin. [● **OBED (pronounced o-BEED): These bacteria are a little bit "pregnant" with phage DNA.**]

B. Recurring infections. Latency in human viruses allows for recurring infections. Latent human viruses include **Herpesviridae** and some **Adenoviridae.** HIV, although inserted, is not truly latent, because it is expressed at a low level continuously unless the patient is being treated with inhibitors.

C. Oncogenesis. Latent viruses may play a role in **human cancers** through:

1. Production of early oncogenic proteins (e.g., HPV)

2. DNA insertion, which results in mutagenesis of a cellular regulatory gene and leads to a loss of growth control

3. Up-regulation, by insertion of a viral transcriptional activator such as HIV's LTR near human genes regulating cell growth.

V. PHENOTYPIC MASKING AND MIXING. When a cell is co-infected with two normal (not defective) and often related viruses, two interesting phenomena may occur. To visualize this, think of one as a red virus (with red capsomers making up the head and red DNA) and the other as a green virus (green capsomers and green DNA).

A. Phenotypic mixing. If the geometry of the heads is very similar, virus may be produced with capsids made up of a mixture of green and red capsomers. Only one kind of DNA (green or red) would be present in each capsid.

B. Phenotypic masking. This occurs when an entirely red capsid forms around a green viral genome; the virus is called a composite virus. The **only way to produce composite viruses** (capsid of one and nucleic acid of another) is for the cell to be infected with the genomes of both viruses. [*Note:* Composite viruses are on the USMLE Step 1 exam to test whether you know that the nucleic acid directs the production of progeny viruses, and that the host cell range is determined by the outer glycoproteins or proteins.]

VI. TRANSFECTION. In the lab, naked viral DNA or positive RNA can be used to infect human cells in culture and initiate viral infection. This is called **transfection.**

VII. VIRUSES AS VECTORS. Viruses circulate in the body, bind to specific cell receptors, and trigger viral uptake and subsequent release of the nucleic acid inside specific cell types. These viral activities are useful to genetic engineers, who create **viral vectors** to deliver genes to repair specific cell types. The needed gene is inserted into the viral vector, which is modified so the viral vector is unable to replicate. Delivery of genes via viral vectors is not without problems (such as the production of viral neutralizing antibodies), but it shows promise in **gene repair** and also in **delivery of drug-producing genes** to specific cells such as brain tumor cells.

IV
Fungi

26

Fungal Basics

I. FUNGAL CHARACTERISTICS. Fungi (**molds, yeasts,** and **mushrooms**) are eukaryotic organisms. Fungal cells have **two major chemical differences from human cells:**

A. Ergosterol, not cholesterol, is the major fungal membrane sterol. Many selectively toxic antifungal agents exploit this difference.

1. Imidazole inhibits synthesis of ergosterol.

2. Amphotericin B and **nystatin** cause cellular leakage after binding to ergosterol.

B. Fungi have **complex carbohydrate and glycoprotein cell walls** (notably chitin, glucans, and mannans), which are potential drug targets and which stain with **calcofluorwhite fluorescent stain.** (Human cells do not fluoresce.)

II. FUNGAL STRUCTURES. Fungi consist of filaments (**hyphae**) or single-celled budding organisms (**yeasts**); some (**dimorphic**) **species** can convert from hyphal forms to yeast forms.

A. Hyphae (filamentous cells) grow to form a mat called a **mycelium.** (On surfaces, the fluffy growth is called a **mold** or aerial mycelium.) There is also a subsurface or vegetative mycelium which penetrates organic substrate to break down and absorb nutrients. **Hyphae grow apically.** Hyphae also make up fruiting bodies that we call mushrooms.

1. Nonseptate hyphae lack cross walls (septations), are broad (7–15 μm wide) and irregular, and branch at obtuse angles. *Mucor* and *Rhizopus* are nonseptate.

2. Septate hyphae have **regular cross walls** and are more uniform in width (2–5 μm in diameter). Most hyphae are septate and colorless (**hyaline**); some genera's hyphae are dark (**dematiaceous**), usually brown to gray.

B. Yeasts are oval to spherical cells that replicate by budding.

C. Dimorphic fungi are generally found at room temperature or in the environment as filamentous fungi (🌡 cold/mold) but grow in the body as yeast or yeastlike form. Important **dimorphic fungi** are *Histoplasma, Blastomyces, Coccidioides,* and *Sporothrix.*

D. Pseudohyphae are formed by *Candida albicans* when buds remain attached and elongate; they look like hyphae with constrictions at each cell-cell juncture. When incubated at 37°C (98°F) in rich medium, *Candida albicans'* yeast cells produce sproutlike projections called **germ tubes** as part of the conversion to hyphal forms. *Candida albicans* colonizes surfaces primarily with yeast forms; when it invades, yeasts, pseudohyphae, and true hyphae are seen.

III. FUNGAL SPORULATION. Most medically important fungi sporulate. **Spore types (all asexual)** include the following:

A. Blastoconidia are the buds on yeasts.

B. Conidia are asexual spores borne on the outside of sporulating hyphae. Some fungi have both macroconidia (slightly larger or multicellular) and microconidia.

C. Endospores (produced by *Coccidioides immitis*) are formed inside large spherical structures (spherules) in tissues.

D. Arthroconidia (arthrospores) are formed by fragmentation of hyphae.

IV. FUNGAL DISEASES

A. **Fungal infection.** Fungal infections (**mycoses**) may start from **overgrowth of normal flora** (generally yeasts or dermatophytes), from **inhalation of fungal spores** (often from a dusty environment), or from **traumatic implantation** of spores into tissues. Fungal infections are particularly **severe in compromised patients,** often disseminating into the bloodstream (**fungemia**).

B. **Fungal toxins**

    1. **Mycotoxicosis** is a poisoning from ingestion of fungal toxins produced in food, most notably the carcinogen **aflatoxin in peanuts.**

    2. **Mycetismus** is illness resulting from ingestion of **toxic mushrooms.**

C. **Allergic reactions**

    1. Allergy to fungi plays a role in allergic **bronchopulmonary aspergillosis** and **farmer's lung.**

    2. **Sick building syndrome** arises from inhalation of volatile fungal toxins and spores, which aggravate allergies.

V. LABORATORY IDENTIFICATION

A. **Fungal culture. Special fungal media** are used.

    1. **Sabouraud's agar,** a standard fungal medium on which most fungi will grow, is used as a clue to fungal infection on exams.

    2. Three media—fungal versions of **blood agar, blood agar with antibiotics** (to inhibit any potential bacterial contaminants), and **blood agar with antibiotics and cycloheximide** (to inhibit fungal contaminants and also some opportunistic or pathogenic fungi—are generally used in culturing suspected systemic fungal infections.

    3. Identification of **fungal isolates** is done by **morphology, biochemical tests** (yeasts), **immunologic tests, or genetic probe.**

B. **Microscopy.** Fungi are visualized in tissues using the following methods:

    1. **Skin scrapings** are dissolved in **10% KOH** to improve ability to see the fungi with a light microscope.

    2. **Calcofluor white** binds to the complex carbohydrate cell wall and lights up the fungi a bright blue white; human cells do not fluoresce.

    3. **Special fungal stains** include the **silver stain** (fungi and basement membranes stain silver), and **periodic acid Schiff (PAS) reaction** (fungi stain hot pink).

    4. **India ink** (used as wet mount medium for CSF sediment) highlights the capsule of

Cryptococcus neoformans, but **has a sensitivity of only 50% so it cannot rule out cryptococcal meningitis. Immunologic methods,** such as latex particle agglutination (LPA) to identify the presence of the capsular polysaccharide antigen in CSF, are much more sensitive than India ink.

    5. Immunofluorescent stains are available for identification of some fungi in tissues.

C. Antibody or antigen detection. Tests for detection of patient antibodies or fungal antigens in body fluids are available. The most critical of the latter group is the detection of Cryptococcal polysaccharide in CSF, as mentioned above.

D. Skin testing. This only demonstrates exposure.

27

Fungi That Cause Skin and Subcutaneous Infections

Malassezia, Dermatophytes (*Trichophyton, Microsporum, Epidermophyton*), *Candida, Sporothrix*

I. *MALASSEZIA FURFUR* is a lipophilic "yeast" found on skin as normal skin flora. It can cause the following disorders:

   A. **Pityriasis versicolor,** which presents as **hypopigmented spots on the chest, back, or both.** Skin scrapings contain clusters of **oval cells and short, curved, septate hyphae.**

   B. **Fungemia** in **premature infants** on intravenous lipid supplements.

II. DERMATOPHYTES

   A. **Three specific genera** of these filamentous fungi infect skin and other keratinized tissues:

   1. *Trichophyton* infects **skin, hair,** and **nails.**

   2. *Microsporum* infects **hair** and **skin.**

   3. *Epidermophyton* infects **nail** and **skin.**

   B. **Reservoir and transmission.** Dermatophytes are **zoophilic, anthropophilic,** or **geophilic. Highly inflammatory** dermatophyte infections (**tineas**) are generally **acquired from animals** (e.g., when setting up milking machines). **Anthropophilic dermatophytes** are spread by **fomites** (e.g., hats, combs, shower room floors) and **direct person-to-person contact.** Most dermatophytes are quite contagious.

   C. **Infections (by location).** Most **tineas** or **ringworms** are named by location: **tinea capitis (hair** and **scalp), tinea barbae (bearded region), tinea corporis (glabrous skin), tinea cruris** or **"jock itch"** (groin and perineal area), and **tinea pedis ("athlete's foot").** The etiologic agents for either tinea cruris or pedis are most commonly *Epidermophyton floccosum* and *Trichophyton* spp. **Favus** or tinea favosa (named for the honeycomb scutula or crusts) is **most serious,** causing **permanent scarring and scalp hair loss.**

   D. **Diagnosis** is either **clinical** or **by microscopy** (KOH mounts of skin, hair, or nail show **arthroconidia and hyphae**).

   E. **Dermatophytid ("id") reaction** is an **allergic response** to circulating dermatophyte antigens released by the dying fungi during antifungal treatment.

III. ***CANDIDA*** is a genus of yeasts. *Candida albicans*, which forms both pseudohyphae and true hyphae in tissue, is common.

    A. **Reservoir and transmission.** Many species of *Candida* are found as normal flora of the mucous membranes and skin. **Predisposing conditions,** such as continuous moisture, occluded skin surfaces, antibiotic use, or diabetes, may cause mucocutaneous overgrowth, resulting in symptoms.

    B. **Infection: Candidiasis.** *Candida* spp. infections range from minor but painful **mucocutaneous lesions** to major problems such as **septicemia or cerebritis** in immunocompromised patients (see Chapter 29). **Pain** and erythema are due to the water-soluble cytotoxin, which damages the skin or mucous membranes.

        1. **Diaper rash** and **yeast vaginitis** are characterized by pain and erythema with a sharp margin between affected and normal skin.

        2. **Thrush** is characterized by a "cheesy" white coating of the oral mucosa with a painful erythematous base.

IV. ***SPOROTHRIX SCHENCKII*** is a dimorphic fungus.

    A. **Reservoir and transmission.** *S. schenckii* grows on a wide variety of **plants** as a filamentous fungus. When it is traumatically implanted into human tissues, the organism converts into a **cigar-shaped yeast.** The implantation may involve **thorns,** floral wire, or slivers; commonly involved plants include roses, plum trees, or sphagnum moss.

    B. **Infection.** Sporotrichosis is commonly called **rose gardener's disease.** There may be **solitary subcutaneous lesions** at the trauma site (usually on extremities), or there may be lesions along the **lymphatics (lymphocutaneous sporotrichosis),** with lymph nodes farther away from the trauma progressively less involved.

    C. **Treatment. Oral potassium iodide** (no antifungal activity) helps break down the tissue response, so that the immune system cells can get in to kill the *Sporothrix.* **Itraconazole** is also used.

28

Thermally Dimorphic Fungi that Cause Fungal Pneumonia and Systemic Fungal Diseases

Histoplasma, Coccidioides, Blastomyces

I. INTRODUCTION. *Histoplasma, Coccidioides,* and *Blastomyces* are the **major systemic fungal pathogens** in the U.S. Some **generalizations** can be made about all three genera:

A. All are **thermally dimorphic.**

B. Infection starts with **inhalation of spores** from an environmental source, often in "dust." Infection is **not transmitted human to human.**

C. *Histoplasma, Blastomyces,* and *Coccidioides* cause **asymptomatic or acute self-resolving fungal pneumonias** in 95% of cases. The rest (5%) become chronic or disseminate to other tissues.

D. Any of these infections, which heal without treatment, **may reactivate later** under immunocompromising conditions.

II. *HISTOPLASMA CAPSULATUM*

A. Characteristics. *Histoplasma capsulatum* has **no capsule.**

1. **Environmental form.** In the environment, *H. capsulatum* is **filamentous fungus** with small microconidia and large **tuberculate macroconidia** (spherical with short fingerlike projections).

2. **Tissue form.** *H. capsulatum* is a **facultative intracellular fungus** seen as a small oval budding yeast (2–4μ) inside cells of the RES.

B. Reservoir and transmission. *H. capsulatum* is associated with **bird- and bat-enriched soil.** The major endemic areas are the **Ohio, Mississippi, and Missouri River beds.** Typical exposure comes from spore inhalation during dusty activities like **cave exploring,** demolition work, or cleaning old **chicken coops.**

C. Disease: Histoplasmosis

1. **Primary histoplasmosis** ranges from asymptomatic to acute self-resolving **fungal pneumonia,** known as the **fungus flu.** Symptoms generally are **cough, fever, malaise, weakness, chest pain, headache, myalgia, chills, nausea, anorexia, and weight loss.** Radiographs in sicker patients show pulmonary infiltrates, with **hilar lymphadenopathy** being common. Lesions have a tendency to calcify.

2. **Systemic infections** occur in **immunocompromised patients,** including AIDS patients. Some are recrudescences of earlier "healed" infections. **Mucocutaneous lesions** (oral or genital) are common in patients with disseminated disease.

D. **Laboratory identification.** Diagnostic suspicion should arise if the patient has pneumonia but has not responded to antibacterial drugs *and* has had **exposure to a dusty environment 1–2 weeks earlier** in the endemic area. Sputum is rarely positive for yeasts, but **Giemsa-stained smears and cultures** of peripheral blood, bone marrow, or urine may be positive for *H. capsulatum.* A fourfold increase in serum antibody titers from acute to convalescent stage is diagnostic.

III. *COCCIDIOIDES IMMITIS*

A. Characteristics

   1. **Environmental form.** *C. immitis* grows in sand as **hyphal filaments** that develop into **arthroconidia.**

   2. **Tissue form.** Inhaled arthroconidia develop into **spherules** (30–60 μ), which produce **endospores** (2–5 μ) internally.

B. **Reservoir and transmission.** *C. immitis* is found in **desert sand in the southwestern U.S.** Airborne arthroconidia are inhaled when the sand is disturbed.

C. Disease: Coccidioidomycosis

   1. **Primary coccidioidomycosis (Valley fever)** ranges from **asymptomatic infection to self-limited fungal pneumonia.** It is most common in children and newcomers to the endemic area. Symptomatic cases present with **cough, fever, and dull chest pain,** along with **flulike symptoms,** resembling any atypical pneumonia. **Erythema nodosum** is a good prognostic sign.

   2. **Disseminated form.** Coccidioidomycosis disseminates more commonly in racial groups with certain HLA types (particularly **African Americans** and **Filipinos**), in **women** in the **third trimester of pregnancy,** and in **immunocompromised patients.** It most commonly disseminates to skin, subcutaneous tissue, bones, joints, or **meninges.**

D. **Laboratory identification.** Incubation is about 4 weeks. **Cultures are hazardous.** Sputum, urine, or bronchial washings may show spherules. A fourfold increase in serum antibody titers from acute to convalescent stage is diagnostic.

IV. *BLASTOMYCES DERMATITIDIS*

A. Characteristics

   1. The **environmental form is hyphae with conidia** arising off short, lateral "stalks."

   2. The **tissue form** is a **large** (8–15 μ) yeast with a **broad-based bud** (i.e., the juncture between the cells is wide) **and a thick, double refractile cell wall.**

B. **Reservoir and transmission.** *Blastomyces* is found in nearly the same geographic region as *Histoplasma,* plus the mid-Atlantic region of the U.S. and northern Minnesota. Environmental association is uncertain but is probably **rotting wood.** Conidia are inhaled.

C. **Disease: Blastomycosis.** This fungal pneumonia is less common than histoplasmosis but more likely to have an indolent onset. It is also less likely to self-resolve and more likely, when it does disseminate, to involve skin and bone.

D. **Laboratory identification.** Cultures are generally done by reference labs. Biopsy specimens examined by microscopy may show large yeast with a wide, budding base and a double, refractile wall. (◐ **Blasto**: **b**road-**b**ased **b**udding yeasts with **b**ig [thick] **wall.**)

29

Opportunistic Fungi

Aspergillus, Candida, Cryptococcus, Mucor, Rhizopus, Absidia, Pneumocystis

I. **INTRODUCTION.** The major opportunistic fungi are monomorphic except some species of *Candida*. The opportunists are either fairly common environmental fungi of low virulence or normal epithelial or mucous membrane flora (*Candida*).

II. ***ASPERGILLUS FUMIGATUS*** is a **monomorphic hyphal fungus** with **dichotomously branching hyphae** having **acute (< 45°) angles** and small (2–3.5 μ), airborne conidia.

   A. **Reservoir and transmission.** Fungi of the genus *Aspergillus* are ubiquitous as major recyclers and so are found in and on almost any moldy organic material (food, ceiling tiles that have been wet, compost, and so on). Inhaled airborne conidia of *Aspergillus fumigatus* are small enough to reach the alveoli. In normal hosts, spores are removed by the mucociliary elevator, or their growth is controlled by macrophages and neutrophils.

   B. Diseases

   1. **Allergic bronchopulmonary aspergillosis** occurs in people with asthma or allergies.

   2. **Fungus balls** grow in preexisting lung cavities, but hyphae do not penetrate the tissue. Disease is characterized by cough, sometimes accompanied by hemoptysis and high IgE.

   3. **Invasive aspergillosis** occurs under conditions of severe neutropenia, chronic granulomatous disease, cystic fibrosis, and burns. Nasal colonization or direct inhalation of large numbers of spores leads to pneumonia. *A. fumigatus* may spread to the brain by direct extension from nares or by hematogenous spread. In burn patients, *Aspergillus* may also disseminate from cellulitis.

III. ***CANDIDA (CANDIDA ALBICANS).*** *Candida* spp. are **yeasts;** a few, like **Candida albicans,** also produce **pseudohyphae and true hyphae in tissues.**

   A. **Reservoir and transmission.** *Candida* spp. are found as **normal mucocutaneous flora** but, under certain conditions, may overgrow *and* invade.

   B. Diseases: Candidiasis

   1. **Oral thrush** occurs in premature infants, patients on antibiotics, and immunocompromised hosts. Oral thrush may progress to esophagitis, then gastritis, and ultimately, through bowel defects, to septicemia.

2. Perlèche (soreness in the mouth angles) suggests malnutrition.

3. Endocarditis (with transient septicemias) occurs in IV drug abusers or people with indwelling catheters.

4. Cerebritis may occur in immunocompromised hosts.

C. Laboratory diagnosis. Microscopy is used to look for pseudohyphae, true hyphae, and budding yeast cells. Sterile sites such as blood are cultured and then **cultures** are speciated using **germ tube formation** and **chemical tests.**

D. Treatment. Mucocutaneous infections with *Candida* spp. can be treated with oral or topical nystatin, which is not absorbed.

IV. *CRYPTOCOCCUS* is a monomorphic yeast that generally has a **generous polysaccharide capsule.**

A. Reservoir and transmission. The environmental source is **soil enriched with pigeon droppings.**

B. Diseases

   1. Acute pulmonary infections may be quite common but are usually asymptomatic except in **pigeon breeders,** presumably because of heavy exposure.

   2. Cryptococcal meningitis is the dominant meningitis of **AIDS patients** and is also seen in **patients with cancer** (e.g., Hodgkin's lymphoma). Pulmonary signs are rarely present.

C. Laboratory identification. Diagnosis of meningitis is commonly made using cerebrospinal fluid (CSF).

   1. The **latex particle agglutination test,** which looks for **capsular antigen in the CSF,** is rapid and sensitive.

   2. Microscopy on **India ink wet mount** of CSF sediment, looking for budding yeasts with **capsular "halos,"** is rapid and useful if the result is positive; however, there is a **negative result in 50% of cryptococcal meningitis cases.**

   3. Cultures of CSF are done, but *C. neoformans* is slow to grow. *C. neoformans* is the **only medically significant, urease-positive yeast.**

V. *MUCOR, RHIZOPUS, ABSIDIA* (ZYGOMYCOTA). The genera of *Rhizopus, Mucor,* and *Absidia* consist of **nonseptate filamentous fungi** (Zygomycota).

A. Reservoir and transmission. These nonseptate filamentous fungi are found in the environment (e.g., **soil,** bread); they produce airborne spores that appear to colonize sinus tracts.

B. Rhinocerebral infection (mucormycosis, phycomycosis, or zygomycosis). The disease presents in **ketoacidotic diabetic patients** and **cancer patients.** Symptoms include **paranasal swelling, mental lethargy,** and **hemorrhagic exudates** in the nose and sometimes the eyes. These organisms are **rapidly invasive** (without respect for barriers) from the sinuses into the **brain,** penetrating vasculature and causing **hemorrhage.**

C. Laboratory identification. Microscopy is used for rapid identification (KOH of necrotic tissues) of **broad, ribbonlike, nonseptate hyphae with about 90° angles on branching.**

D. Treatment includes rapid **debridement** of necrotic tissue, high-dose **amphotericin B,** and, if diabetes is involved, lowering blood glucose. The fatality rate is high.

VI. ***PNEUMOCYSTIS CARINII*** is an obligate extracellular fungus that cannot be grown in the lab. *Pneumocystis* **is now considered a fungus** as a result of **ribotyping**[1] **and other molecular techniques.**

  A. Disease. *Pneumocystis* exposure is quite common, but disease **(an atypical pneumonia)** occurs primarily in **AIDS patients** or in **severely malnourished or premature infants.** The disease presents as an **interstitial pneumonia** which, on X-ray film, may have a **ground-glass appearance.**

  B. Laboratory identification: stains. Lung tissue stained with **H & E** shows **alveoli with a foamy appearance,** sometimes referred to as a **honeycomb** appearance. With **silver** stain, **silver-stained cysts** appear in the center spaces. Silver stain of bronchial alveolar fluid also shows silver-stained cysts.

  C. Treatment. **Trimethoprim/sulfamethoxazole prophylaxis** is used in known HIV positive patients with < 200 CD4+ cells/mm³.

[1]Ribotyping compares ribosomal base sequences, which are very well conserved within groups of related organisms.

V
Parasites

30

Parasite Basics

I. OVERVIEW OF PARASITES. A parasite is an **organism** (from virus to animal) that **lives in or on another organism (the host)** *and* **does some damage to the host in the process.** This chapter and Chapters 31 through 34 discuss animal (protozoan or helminthic) parasites. Animal parasites are **eukaryotic** organisms with **no cell walls,** ranging from **single-celled organisms to large, multicellular worms.** There are several types of parasites:

    A. A **facultative parasite** can live in association with its host or separately.

    B. An **obligate parasite** cannot live free of the host for at least some stage of the life cycle.

    C. A **parasite with a complex life cycle** requires more than one host.

II. HOSTS. A host is an organism that provides nutrition and a place for the parasite to replicate.

    A. A **reservoir host** maintains a parasite and may be the source for human infection. An **essential reservoir host** is one without which the parasite cannot exist (e.g., cats for *Toxoplasma*).

    B. An **intermediate host** either maintains the **asexual stage(s)** of a parasite or allows development of the parasite to proceed only to the **larval stage.**

    C. A **definitive host** is one in which the **adult** or **sexual parasites** develop.

III. VECTORS are biological systems that **spread parasites.**

    A. A **biological vector** (e.g., the *Anopheles* mosquito in malaria) **serves both as a vector and a host** for the **replicative stage** of a parasite.

    B. A **mechanical vector transmits a parasite without being a host** (e.g., flies "tracking" *Chlamydia trachomatis* from one eye to the next).

IV. MAJOR GROUPS OF ANIMAL PARASITES[1]

    A. **Protozoa** are single-celled animals. **Trophozoites** are the more delicate **motile** forms of protozoa. **Cysts,** the **infectious protozoan stage in fecal-oral transmission,** survive in the environment and in stomach acid.

        1. **Amebas** move by pseudopodia. Pathogenic amebas include *Entamoeba histolytica, Naegleria fowleri,* and *Acanthamoeba.*

---

[1]Major groups are considered important for physicians, because antiparasitic agents are often broad enough to be used against a whole group (e.g., an anti-nematode drug).

2. **Flagellates** move by one or more flagella. Pathogens include *Giardia lamblia, Trichomonas vaginalis, Trypanosoma,* and *Leishmania.*

3. **Sporozoans (Apicomplexa)** are obligate intracellular protozoans with complex life cycles and at least two different hosts. Sporozoans include *Plasmodium, Cryptosporidium,* and *Toxoplasma.*

B. **Roundworms (nematodes)** are **round in cross-section,** with tapering ends. (●A nemesis is some one who **bugs** you and is always "a-**round**" you.) Nematodes have separate male and female individuals and well-developed GI tracts. "High-yield" nematodes are *Ascaris* and *Enterobius.*

C. **Flatworms** are flat, multicellular worms. There are two groups:

1. **Trematodes** are also called **flukes.** (●Think: fluke, flutter, tremor, trematode.) Flukes are generally **flat, fleshy, nonsegmented worms.** All trematodes have complex life cycles involving **snails as intermediate hosts** and **water transmission to humans. Schistosomes** are important flukes.

2. **Cestodes** are **tapeworms (segmented flatworms). Cestodes have complex life cycles with at least two hosts.** Intermediate hosts ingest eggs, which develop into larvae in tissue, often resulting in serious disease. Hosts that ingest larvae from infected tissues develop intestinal, adult tapeworms.

V. CHARACTERISTICS OF PARASITIC DISEASE

A. **Symptoms** are generally **proportional to parasite burden** and may be more severe once the individual is sensitized to parasitic components.

B. **Reinfections** may occur. **Autoinfection** (reinfection of the host without the organism going through developmental stages elsewhere) is common with *Strongyloides* and *Enterobius.*

C. **Chronic infections** may occur (e.g., Chagas' disease), with or without overt disease. Some parasites can remain viable in humans for long periods, in some cases throughout a person's life, and may cause periodic disease symptoms.

D. **Immunocompromising conditions** may cause **reactivation** of latent infections (such as toxoplasmosis), **increased susceptibility,** and often **more severe disease.**

E. **Eosinophilia** is sometimes a clue to parasitic disease, although it generally only occurs **during larval worm migration** through the vasculature or tissue.

VI. LABORATORY DIAGNOSTIC METHODS for parasitic infections vary with frequency of infections in a country, and the size and expertise of the laboratory. The more sophisticated tests are often available only in larger reference laboratories.

A. **Microscopic examination** of tissues, blood, and feces (generally following concentration methods) is still used. Worms infecting the GI tract are still mostly identified in the U.S. by microscopic identification of the eggs in feces. **Helminthic eggs** likely to be used as clues in USMLE cases are shown in **Figure 30-1.**

B. **Cultures.** Culture techniques are used to identify some protozoans.

C. **Antigens/antibodies.** Tests demonstrating the presence of antigens for a specific organism are now available for some tissue, blood, and GI tract pathogens. Also, tests demonstrating patient antibody are available for some parasites.

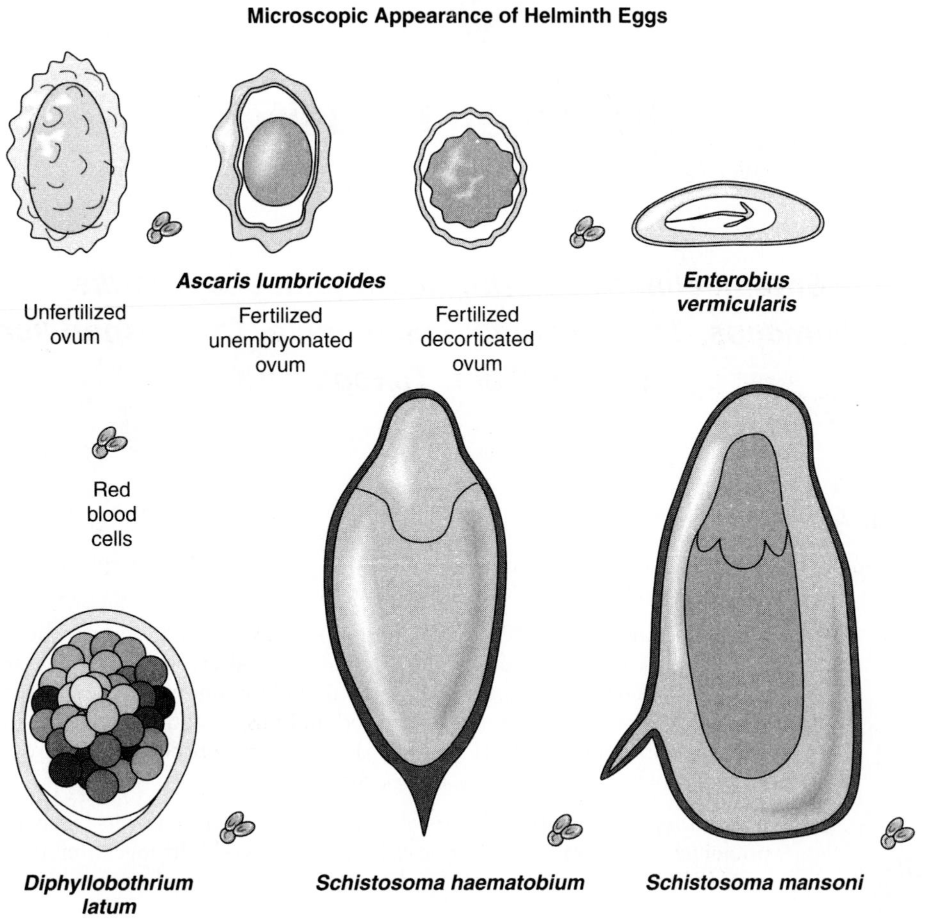

Microscopic Appearance of Helminth Eggs

Ascaris lumbricoides

Unfertilized
ovum

Fertilized
unembryonated
ovum

Fertilized
decorticated
ovum

*Enterobius
vermicularis*

Red
blood
cells

*Diphyllobothrium
latum*

Schistosoma haematobium

Schistosoma mansoni

Figure 30-1.   Common worm eggs and their proportional sizes.

31

Protozoan Parasites

Entamoeba, Naegleria, Acanthamoeba, Giardia, Trichomonas, Trypanosoma, Leishmania, Cryptosporidium, Plasmodium, Toxoplasma

I. AMEBAS

A. *Entamoeba histolytica* is a human pathogen of the **large intestine** spread by **cysts** via the **fecal-oral route** in areas of poor sanitation.

    1. **Disease: amebic dysentery.** Ingested cysts break down to release the ameboid trophozoites, which invade large intestinal mucosal crypts and feed on red cells, causing **flask-shaped ulcers.** Symptoms include **crampy diarrhea** or **dysentery** (abdominal cramps with tenesmus, blood and pus in stools). **Extraintestinal abscesses** (particularly in **liver** and **lung**) are a **common complication of *E. histolytica*.** Inapparent infections also occur.

    2. **Laboratory identification.** *E. histolytica* can be recognized by its **"wagon wheel" nuclei** (sharp central dot with fine chromatin "spokes"). Its **ingestion of red blood cells** (RBCs) distinguishes it from the commensal *Entamoeba coli*, which does not cause disease.

B. *Naegleria*, a free-living ameba found in contaminated **hot water**, infects humans during **swimming or diving.** *Naegleria* causes **primary amebic meningoencephalitis (PAM).** Onset is **rapid**, with headache and fever followed by nausea, vomiting, sensation of constant odd odor or taste, and irrational behavior. There are meningeal, frontal, temporal, and cerebellar signs. **Coma and death are common** within 6 days. On microscopy, the cerebrospinal fluid should show **trophozoites, PMNs, and RBCs.**

C. *Acanthamoeba* is a **free-living ameba** that is probably spread by inhalation. **Diseases** caused by *Acanthamoeba* include:

    1. **Granulomatous amebic meningoencephalitis (GAE) in immunocompromised patients.** GAE has a more **chronic onset** (less fulminant and more benign) than PAM. Symptoms reflect focal lesions. **Spiky trophozoites** are seen in CSF or brain tissue.

    2. **Keratitis.** *Acanthamoeba*-contaminated contact lens saline along with minor eye abrasion can cause keratitis, characterized by **corneal inflammation and pain.**

II. FLAGELLATES

A. *Giardia lamblia* is a distinctive **teardrop-shaped flagellated protozoan with a ventral sucking disk.** Cysts are the infectious form.

1. **Reservoir and transmission.** *Giardia lamblia* is found **worldwide in water** contaminated by **infected beavers, muskrats,** or **poor human sanitation.** Expect cases in **wilderness campers.** Like other diseases with fecal-oral transmission, it can also be transmitted in **day care settings** and by **oral-anal sex.**

2. **Disease: giardiasis.** *Giardia's* **ventral sucking disk attaches** to the **duodenal/jejunal** surface, blocks adsorption, and causes irritation and blunting of microvilli. Symptoms vary from **mild watery diarrhea to malabsorption syndrome** with epigastric pain, **severe abdominal cramping,** flatulence, and **light-colored, fatty stools.**

3. **Laboratory identification.** Because of its attachment, *Giardia* is not seen in the feces of 60% of those infected. *Giardia* **fecal antigen tests** have replaced the string test when microscopy is negative.

B. *Trichomonas vaginalis* is a **sexually transmitted flagellate** with both an **undulating membrane** and a **polar tuft of flagella.** The infectious **trophozoite** has a **contact-dependent cytopathic effect.**

1. **Disease.** Trichomonal vaginitis is characterized by a **malodorous** (fishy), **purulent yellow vaginal discharge** and **erythematous vaginal mucosa.** Dyspareunia, urinary frequency, and dysuria may also be present. **Males are often asymptomatic.**

2. **Laboratory identification.** Wet mounts or antigen detection tests are used.

C. *Trypanosoma brucei rhodesiense* and *T. brucei gambiense* (*T. brucei*) are flagellates spread by the **tsetse fly.**

1. **Disease: trypanosomiasis** or **African sleeping sickness (ASS).** *T. brucei* invade the blood and lymphatics causing **fever, headache, malaise, rash,** and **posterior cervical lymph node enlargement (Winterbottom's sign.)** Sequelae range from spontaneous cure to **invasion of the CNS,** leading to ASS, coma, and death.

2. **Virulence and laboratory identification.** The progressive nature of untreated ASS is due to extreme **antigenic variation of trypanosomal surface glycoproteins** (over 1000 variants), which allows evasion of the immune system. **IgM levels are generally > 4 times normal.** Normal serum IgM levels rule out ASS.

D. *Trypanosoma cruzi* is a flagellate found from **Mexico to South America,** where American trypanosomiasis **(Chagas' disease)** is a significant cause of death.

1. **Reservoir and transmission. Mammals are intermediate hosts** and **reduviid bugs** ("cone-nosed" or "kissing" bugs) **are definitive hosts.** Transmission may be through the **placenta** (causing a high rate of stillbirths), organ transplantation, **blood transfusion** (an increasing problem in the U.S.), or reduviid bugs that defecate as they bite. The infected person scratches, depositing the fecal *T. cruzi* into the wound and producing a painful, indurated ulcer **(chagoma).**

2. **Disease: American trypanosomiasis.** Spread of *T. cruzi* leads to additional chagomas, often **swelling around one eye (Romaña's sign),** variable **high fever,** malaise, lymphadenopathy, and hepatosplenomegaly. Spontaneous cure may occur.
   a. In the **very young,** progressive disease often leads to **meningoencephalitis and death.**
   b. In older children or **adults,** disease is more chronic, causing an **enlarged, flaccid heart** that may cause **sudden death** or, less commonly, **megaesophagus or megacolon.**

3. **Laboratory identification.** Microscopy can reveal the **flagellated trypomastigotes** in blood or **nonmotile amastigotes** in tissue culture; xenodiagnosis, ELISA, and PCR are also available.

E. *Leishmania* species all multiply in and are transmitted by **sandflies.** *Leishmania* infect macrophages of their mammalian hosts. **Leishmanial diseases** vary with species:

  1. *Leishmania donovani* complex causes **visceral leishmaniasis** (kala-azar), invading skin (early), spleen, liver, and bone marrow. Hepatosplenomegaly, anemia, weight loss, and indefinite feeling of unwellness are common. There may be fever, including double (dromedary) or triple **fever peaks** daily.

  2. *Leishmania tropica* complex causes **cutaneous leishmaniasis,** also called **Oriental sore.**

  3. *Leishmania braziliensis* complex causes **mucocutaneous leishmaniasis** and destroys soft tissue of the nose and palate. Bone is not invaded.

III. SPOROZOA. Sporozoans are **intracellular protozoans** with **both sexual and asexual stages,** sometimes in different hosts. Their apical complex structure enables them to invade cells, so they are also called **Apicomplexa.** "High-yield" sporozoa are *Cryptosporidium, Plasmodium,* and *Toxoplasma.*

A. *Cryptosporidium parvum* is found frequently in U.S. **surface waters.** It is not killed by chlorination of water, so it is **removed in drinking water treatment by flocculation or filtration.** It is usually acquired by swimming in or drinking untreated water.

  1. **Disease.** Cryptosporidiosis is a **self-limiting diarrhea** in **healthy** people. In **immunocompromised** people, it causes **chronic diarrhea** with **abdominal pain, fever, and anorexia resulting in weight loss** and death. (There is no proven efficacious drug treatment.)

  2. **Laboratory identification** is via **microscopy** (finding **acid-fast oocysts** in feces or intestinal biopsies) or **fecal antigen tests.**

B. *Plasmodium* species are sporozoans that cause **malaria, the most common fatal infectious disease** in the world. Most malaria is acquired in the tropics or subtropics; rare **"airport malaria"** is acquired from infected mosquitoes traveling on airplanes.

  1. **Reservoir and transmission.** Four species of *Plasmodium* cause malaria. A general life cycle is shown in **Figure 31-1** and outlined below.

  a. *Anopheles* mosquitoes inject sporozoites that infect only the **liver parenchymal cells** and develop into **schizonts** containing thousands of daughter cells, called **merozoites.**

  b. In *P. ovale* and *P. vivax* only, a second liver form also develops called **hypnozoites (sleeping forms),** which remain **quiescent** for years. **Primaquine is required to kill hypnozoites;** if not used, a recurrence of symptoms (**relapse**) comes from the **liver hypnozoites.** (🔵 It's not "<u>ov</u>er" if you treat <u>o</u>vale or <u>vi</u>vax malaria only with chloroquine.)

  c. Liver schizonts lyse, releasing **merozoites,** which **infect only red blood cells** (not liver).

  (1) *P. vivax* and *P. ovale* infect only reticulocytes (< 2% of the RBCs).

  (2) *P. malariae* infects only senescent red cells.

  (3) *P. falciparum* infects all RBCs, resulting in **prominent anemia** and **RBC** surface changes (knobs), which cause **endothelial adherence** with decreased microcirculation, DIC, and cerebral malaria. Duffy antigen-negative RBCs are resistant to merozoite invasion.

  d. **RBC stages. Trophozoites** (ring stages) develop into schizonts with more merozoites. Release of large numbers of erythrocytic merozoites and **hemoglobin breakdown products** at one time results in the typical **malarial fever paroxysm.** Some infected red cells produce and release **gametocytes.**

Plasmodium Life Cycle

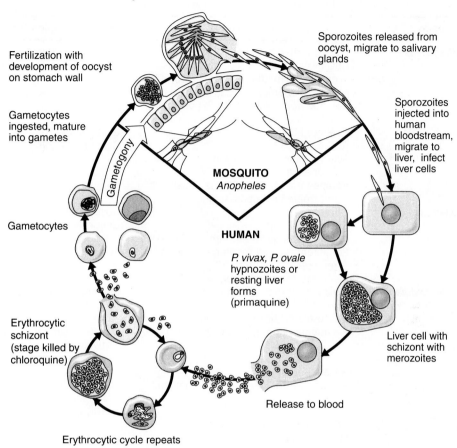

Fertilization with development of oocyst on stomach wall

Sporozoites released from oocyst, migrate to salivary glands

Gametocytes ingested, mature into gametes

Sporozoites injected into human bloodstream, migrate to liver, infect liver cells

Gametogony

MOSQUITO
Anopheles

Gametocytes

HUMAN

P. vivax, P. ovale hypnozoites or resting liver forms (primaquine)

Erythrocytic schizont (stage killed by chloroquine)

Liver cell with schizont with merozoites

Release to blood

Erythrocytic cycle repeats

Figure 31-1. General life cycle of the *Plasmodium* species that cause malaria.

   e. **The sexual cycle** begins with **ingestion of the gametocytes** by an *Anopheles* mosquito.

2. **Disease symptoms** are species-dependent (**Table 31-1**). Malaria always starts with an **influenzalike prodrome** followed by periodic paroxysms. **Paroxysms are shaking chills,** a **pale cyanotic** appearance, and fever, followed by a **flushed, hot stage** with **agitation, disorientation, severe frontal headache,** and **limbic** pain. Sweating follows the hot stage, which ends in **severe exhaustion and sleep.** Patients are often asymptomatic when they wake up.

3. **Laboratory identification** of *Plasmodium* is by microscopic examination of (see Table 31-1).

4. **Prophylaxis and treatment. Chloroquine kills only erythrocytic stages.** Thus, malarial prophylaxis is continued for 4 weeks after leaving a malarious region; this allows all liver schizonts to convert to RBC forms and be killed. If *P. vivax* or *P.*

Table 31-1
Major Distinguishing Characteristics of Plasmodia

Species	Disease	Microscopic Clues
Plasmodium vivax	Benign tertian malaria RBC cycle 44–48 hr Average plasmodia per mm^3 = 20,000 Moderate anemia Relapse from hypnozoites is possible if not treated with primaquine.	Schüffner's granules May have two ring forms
Plasmodium ovale	Ovale or benign tertian malaria RBC cycle 48 hr Average plasmodia per mm^3 = 9,000 Mild anemia Relapse from hypnozoites is possible if not treated with primaquine.	Enlarged oval red cells Schüffner's granules
Plasmodium malariae	Quartan malaria RBC cycle 72 hr Average plasmodia per mm^3 = 6,000 Persistent <u>red</u> <u>c</u>ell forms may lead to <u>rec</u>rudescence up to 30 yr later. Moderate to severe anemia	Rosette schizonts Uniformly round infected RBCs
Plasmodium falciparum	Malignant tertian malaria RBC cycle 48 hr or continuous Plasmodia per mm^3 = 50,000–500,000 Severe anemia Infected RBCs adhere to endothelium. CNS involvement Medical emergency	Multiply infected red cells (1–3/cell) Double "signet ring" forms (two chromatin dots per ring) Schizonts rarely seen in peripheral blood due to RBC adherence Crescent-shaped gametes

ovale infection is diagnosed, treatment with primaquine is added to the standard chloroquine treatment. **Drug resistance is a problem in P. *falciparum.***

C. *Toxoplasma gondii*

1. **Reservoir and transmission (Figure 31-2). Sexual stages** occur *only in cats* (definitive hosts). All vertebrates serve as intermediate hosts. Rodents that eat cat feces contaminate fields, infecting cattle, sheep, pigs, and other animals. **Human exposures** occur through ingestion of **undercooked meat,** exposure to **cat feces,** or **transplacental transfer.** In the initial infection, *Toxoplasma* creates **cysts that may remain viable for years,** producing **long-lasting antibody titers** and potential for later relapse under immunocompromising conditions. Antibodies in women infected prior to pregnancy prevent transplacental transfer. In **antibody-negative women infected during pregnancy,** the baby may be infected.

2. Disease: human toxoplasmosis

   a. **Healthy adults** generally have benign **asymptomatic or mononucleosis-like** infections with **persistent cysts.**

   b. In antibody-positive AIDS patients whose CD4+ cells are less than 100/µl

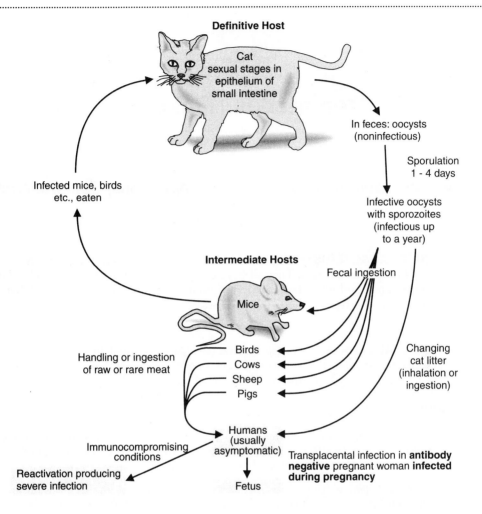

Figure 31-2.   Life cycle of *Toxoplasma gondii*. Infection during pregnancy can cause toxoplasmosis in the baby.

(with no prophylaxis), *toxoplasmosis* may **reactivate,** leading to **retinochoroiditis** and **focal CNS lesions.**

   c. In **fetuses,** infections range from **asymptomatic to severe (encephalomyelitis with calcifications, retinochoroiditis,** and either **hydrocephalus** or **micro-cephaly).** Asymptomatic but infected neonates (usually infected in the third trimester) may develop **retinochoroiditis** if not identified and treated.

3. **Laboratory identification** is made via **serology.**

32

Trematodes (Flukes)

Fasciolopsis, Clonorchis, Fasciola, Paragonimus, Schistosoma

I. FLUKE CHARACTERISTICS. Flukes are **highly organized, nonsegmented flatworms** with an **incomplete GI tract.** They **all have complex life cycles involving snails as intermediate hosts** and **water transmission to humans** or other definitive hosts. Characteristics of the two types of flukes (**separate sexes and hermaphroditic**) are outlined in Table 32-1.

II. INTESTINAL FLUKES. *Fasciolopsis buski* (the giant intestinal fluke) is found in Asia and India. Human infection occurs when **cysts on water plants** (bamboo sprouts, water chestnuts) **are ingested.** Diarrhea is a symptom of infection.

III. LIVER FLUKES

A. *Clonorchis sinensis* (the Chinese liver fluke) is transmitted by **raw or undercooked freshwater fish.** In infected humans, the adult worms localize in distal parts of the **biliary tree,** sometimes living more than 30 years.

B. *Fasciola hepatica* (the sheep liver fluke) is cosmopolitan in **sheep-raising areas.** (🐑 Add "S," making it **sh**epatica, to remind you of sheep.) Transmission is by ingestion of metacercariae on **watercress or other aquatic plants.**

Table 32-1
Two Major Types of Flukes (Trematodes): Characteristics, Transmission, and Diagnosis

Type	Transmission	Diagnostic Stage
Schistosomes— **Separate sexes**	Larvae (in water) penetrate human skin. Genus: *Schistosoma*	Eggs with spines (no operculum)
Tissue flukes— **Hermaphroditic**	Encysted larvae are eaten in raw or undercooked food. Genus (infected food): *Fasciola* (watercress) *Fasciolopsis* (water chestnuts, water plants) *Paragonimus* (crab) *Clonorchis* (fish)	Operculated eggs ("hinged lid")

IV. LUNG FLUKE. *Paragonimus westermani* is found in **India, Asia, and Africa.** Human infection starts with ingestion of infected **shellfish. Adult flukes** in the **lungs** cause fever, cough and hemoptysis. **Eggs** are expelled in sputum and feces.

V. BLOOD FLUKES (SCHISTOSOMES)

   A. Shared schistosomal characteristics

   1. The **male** is flat but folds in ventrally to hold the **female** (longer, slender, and rounder) in permanent copulation.

   2. Schistosomal **larvae (found in water)** penetrate human skin, causing early **dermatitis. Adult flukes** mature in **abdominal veins.**

   3. Schistosomal **egg spines** (see Figure 30-1) play an important role in **disease and spread.** Granulomas may form around the eggs. The physical irritation from the spine and egg enzymes erodes the venules and underlying tissues, liberating the eggs into the intestine or bladder lumen.

   4. Schistosomiasis is one of the most common infectious causes of death in the world. About 150 million people are infected; there are approximately 1 million deaths per year, primarily among heavily infected native people.

   B. *Schistosoma mansoni* (seen in **Africa, Middle East, S. America,** and the **Caribbean**) causes **intestinal schistosomiasis.** Adult flukes mature in the mesenteric venules. Patients may be asymptomatic or have diarrhea, abdominal pain, and hepatosplenomegaly. **Eggs with lateral spines in stool** are diagnostic.

   C. *Schistosoma japonicum* (found in the **Far East** in **rice paddies**) also causes **intestinal schistosomiasis,** but eggs are more frequently **carried in the circulation to distant sites** (often to the choroid plexus and venules around the spinal cord).

   D. *Schistosoma haematobium* (seen in **Africa and the Middle East**) causes **vesicular schistosomiasis.** Adult flukes reproduce in bladder veins. **Eggs** (having a **terminal spine**) are trapped in the **bladder venules;** they cause granulomas and erosion, resulting in urgency, frequency, dysuria, and hematuria. **Bladder carcinoma** in Egypt has a high association with chronic schistosomiasis.

   E. Schistosomes that normally infect aquatic birds and animals may cause **schistosomal dermatitis (swimmer's itch)** in humans. They die after penetrating the skin in humans.

VI. TREATMENT OF FLUKE INFECTION. Praziquantel is used to treat all trematode infections except swimmer's itch, which is treated with calamine.

33

Cestodes (Tapeworms)

Taenia, Diphyllobothrium, Echinococcus

I. CESTODE BASICS

A. Definition. Cestodes are **segmented flatworms.** Adults have three types of segments: the **scolex** (head); the **neck region,** which produces numerous **proglottids;** and the **strobila,** the linearly arranged proglottids that make up the major part of the worm. **Each proglottid contains both a female and a male genital tract.** Mature distal proglottids produce fertilized eggs.

B. Life cycle. Cestode life cycles are complex. Some cestodes have early larval and late larval forms, so there may be more than one intermediate host in addition to the definitive host. Because of wanderings of larval forms and their development in tissues, **disease is more serious in the intermediate host(s).** In the definitive host, the adult tapeworms are in the GI tract, where they may be asymptomatic or simply cause vague abdominal discomfort, unless there is a heavy worm burden.

II. INTESTINAL TAPEWORMS (HUMANS AS DEFINITIVE HOST)

A. *Taenia solium* (pork tapeworm) and *Taenia saginata* (beef tapeworm). When larval forms (cysticerci) in undercooked pork, game, or beef are ingested by humans, adult tapeworms (growing to **several meters long**) develop in the intestine. **Thick-walled spherical, dark brown eggs in the feces are diagnostic.** (*Note:* Trichinella is the pork roundworm.)

B. *Diphyllobothrium latum* (the broad fish tapeworm)

1. **Description. Proglottids** of *D. latum* are **more broad than long** (thus the nickname); the adult tapeworms can grow to 10 meters. The tapeworm is found in **fish in cool freshwater lakes.** It has largely been eliminated from Minnesota and Michigan lakes, formerly the major endemic area in the U.S.

2. **Infection.** Ingestion of infected **undercooked or pickled fish** can lead to largely **asymptomatic infections of the small intestine.** *Diphyllobothrium latum* outcompetes the host for vitamin B_{12}. **Macrocytic hyperchromic anemia may occur through B_{12} deficiency** if the tapeworm attaches high in the jejunum.

III. TISSUE CESTODES (HUMANS AS INTERMEDIATE HOST). If humans ingest either tapeworm eggs or early larvae, they may serve as the intermediate host to early or later larvae, respectively. The larvae develop in the tissues and so have **more serious consequences than intestinal tapeworms.** Several diseases may develop:

A. Cysticercosis. If humans ingest **embryonated eggs of _Taenia solium_** (pork tapeworm) from other human fecal waste, the hatched **larvae exit the intestinal wall** to the bloodstream **and may infect any tissue,** most seriously the **eye** (with visual loss) or the **brain.** The kidney bean–shaped cysticerci calcify and can be seen on X-ray films.

B. Sparganosis. If **tiny crustaceans carrying the very earliest larval forms of _Diphyllobothrium latum_** (broad fish tapeworm) **are ingested** with water, the later larval form **(sparganum)** develops in the human (generally **in subcutaneous tissues**).

C. Hydatid cyst disease. Accidental human ingestion of the embryonated eggs of _Echinococcus granulosis_ from canine fecal contamination results in the growth of the embryo into a **hydatid cyst.** This space-filling structure, which can grow **up to 20 cm in diameter** after a decade, is most commonly located in lung or liver. The hydatid cyst contains **infectious protoscoleces,** hydatid sand, and an **anaphylatoxin. Treatment** is with albendazole followed by aspiration of the cyst contents and subsequent injection of scolecidal fluid; this treatment is replacing very careful surgical removal. **Deworming of sheep dogs** with praziquantel every 6 weeks has reduced the incidence.

D. Alveolar hydatid cyst (from _Echinococcus multilocularis_) is similar to hydatid cyst disease, except that multiple smaller cysts bud out, producing a structure that resembles alveoli.

34

Nematodes (Roundworms)

Enterobius, Ascaris, Trichuris, Trichinella, Strongyloides, Ancylostoma, Necator, Wuchereria, Brugia, Loa loa, Onchocerca, Dracunculus

I. NEMATODE BASICS

A. Definition. Nematodes **are roundworms with unsegmented bodies. Humans** are a **definitive host.** Nematodes have **separate sexes** (males are generally smaller) and produce large numbers of eggs (up to 1 million per female in some species). Larvae develop through a series of molts, some requiring warm, moist soil. The third-stage larva **(filariform)** is generally the **infectious nematode form** for humans, except for a few cases where eggs are ingested.

B. Infection. Migration in vasculature produces **eosinophilia.** Severity of symptoms depends on worm burden, previous sensitization, and nutritional status of the infected individual. Previous infection does not prevent reinfection. Some worms are long-lived.

C. Overview of intestinal nematodes. Some forms are ingested (*Enterobius*, *Ascaris*, *Trichuris*, *Trichinella*— 🔵 EAT²), whereas others penetrate skin (*Strongyloides*, *Ancylostoma*, *Necator*— 🔵 S[k]AN). Intestinal roundworms usually mature in the **small intestine,** where most adults attach by anterior oral hooks or cutting plates. They cause disease by **blood loss, irritation,** and **allergy.** Their invasiveness spreads the roundworm larvae which may result in **secondary bacterial infections.**

D. Overview of tissue nematodes. They are spread by **mosquitoes** (*Wuchereria* and *Brugia*) or **biting flies** (*Loa loa* and *Onchocerca*), except for *Dracunculus*, which is ingested in contaminated drinking water. Adult tissue nematodes produce symptoms due to irritation or inflammation from nematode secretions or components in the lymphatics, leading to **lymphangitis** and, ultimately, **elephantiasis** of genitalia or limbs.

E. 🔵 **Mnemonic. <u>NEMA²T³ODES</u>**

<u>N</u>ecator (U.S. hookworms)
<u>E</u>nterobius (pinworms)
<u>M</u>os<u>q</u>uito borne: <u>W</u>uchereria and Br<u>u</u>gia
<u>A</u>²—<u>A</u>scaris and <u>A</u>ncylostoma
<u>T</u>³—<u>T</u>richuris, <u>T</u>richinella, and <u>T</u>oxocara
<u>O</u>nchocerca (river blindness)
<u>D</u>racunculus (Guinea worm, nearly eradicated)
<u>E</u>ye worm (*Loa loa*)
<u>S</u>trongyloides (threadworm)

II. INTESTINAL NEMATODES

A. *Ascaris lumbricoides.* This **large nematode** (adults up to 0.5 × 35 cm) is the **most common roundworm,** and also the **most common parasite,** in the world (approximately 1 billion people are infected). In areas of poor sanitation nearly everyone is infected, often with heavy worm burdens.

1. Life cycle. *Ascaris* **eggs are ingested;** larvae hatch, exit the duodenal wall, and migrate through the vasculature into the liver, heart, and lungs. In the lungs they burst out into the alveoli, causing a **pneumonitis.** As with other worm migrations through the vasculature, **eosinophils and IgE levels may be elevated.** Molting, migrating, and being carried by cough, the larvae eventually reach the esophagus and enter the GI tract again. There they mature in the **small intestines** and the females lay eggs.

2. Disease: ascariasis. Adult ascarids do not attach but maintain their position in the intestines by **motility.** Infected people with low worm burdens are often asymptomatic. In children with heavy worm burdens, the **worms may tangle and produce an intestinal blockage.** Increased worm migration is seen with **fever, anesthesia, or antibiotic use** and may result in **blockage of bile ducts or appendix,** or in migration up the esophagus or into the gallbladder.

B. *Enterobius vermicularis* (pinworm) is the **most common roundworm infection in the U.S.**

1. Life cycle and infection. *Enterobius* infection begins with ingestion of eggs in household dust from contaminated clothing or bedding. Adult female pinworms (up to 0.5 inches long) migrate out to perianal areas and lay eggs, causing **intense perianal itching. Autoinfection** occurs from perianal scratching and then putting fingers in the mouth.

2. Diagnosis. A tongue depressor with scotch tape (sticky side out) has been used for a perianal sampler. A plastic paddle/slide with one sticky surface is now available for obtaining samples (this is generally done at home).

C. Hookworms. *Necator americanus* (New World hookworms endemic in southeast U.S.) and *Ancylostoma duodenale* (Old World hookworms) thrive in warm, humid climates.

1. Life cycle and disease. Eggs in feces deposited into soil develop into filariform larvae, which attach between the toes of **bare feet** and **penetrate skin.** They migrate through the bloodstream into alveoli, causing a **pneumonitis.** Then they migrate up the trachea or are coughed up and swallowed, reentering the GI tract and attaching to the small intestine. Repeated infections lead to allergy at entry points **("ground itch")** and more severe pneumonitis. Infections are commonly **chronic,** leading to **weight loss,** microcytic hypochromic **anemia,** and **fatigue,** particularly if nutrition is poor.

2. Prevention is by wearing shoes and/or improving sanitation.

D. *Strongyloides stercoralis* (threadworm) is found in **tropical and subtropical areas** (e.g., southeastern United States) in the soil, from human fecal contamination. Like hookworms, *S. stercoralis* **penetrates feet** and migrates through the vasculature. Unlike hookworms, **some larvae** develop that **reinvade the intestinal wall** and begin an **autoinfection** without leaving the human host to develop in soil. Thus, untreated people may be infected for years.

E. *Trichuris trichiura* (whipworm) is found in the **tropics** in areas of poor sanitation. **Eggs are ingested,** larvae develop in the small intestine, and adults attach in the large intestine. **Trichuriasis** is frequently asymptomatic; in heavier infections, it causes **ab-**

dominal pain with mucoid or bloody diarrhea, tenesmus (sometimes resulting in rectal prolapse), and weight loss. It worsens poor nutrition.

F. *Trichinella spiralis* (pork roundworm) has **both intestinal and tissue stages** in humans.

    1. **Intestinal stage.** Larvae are ingested in **pork or wild game** (e.g., bear or deer) and develop into adults. Early symptoms are **nausea and abdominal pain with vomiting and diarrhea, fever, and headache.**

    2. **Tissue stage.** Female worms burrow to lay eggs in submucosa (so there are **no eggs in stools**). Larvae hatch and migrate into the bloodstream, then out into striated muscle, causing degenerative and inflammatory changes in the fibers. The **coiled larvae may calcify.** The symptoms of the circulation and tissue stages generally come 2 to 8 weeks after the GI symptoms and include **high fever, eosinophilia (10%–90%), myalgia, periorbital edema, conjunctival and subungual (splinter) hemorrhages, and urticarial rash.**

III. TISSUE NEMATODES: FILARIAL WORMS. All are **transmitted** to humans **via an arthropod bite.** None is significant in the U.S. Only the scientific name, common name, and the vector are "high-yield" information.

    A. *Onchocerca volvulus* (spread by the *Simulium* blackfly) causes **river blindness,** one of the WHO's six most harmful infectious diseases. Subcutaneous nodules around adult nematodes are prominent early. Sensitization of the human host to the filariae, which then migrate through the body, leads to **allergic-toxic reaction,** including abnormal **skin and subcutaneous tissue reactions,** and **eye reactions leading to blindness.**

    B. *Loa loa* (eye worm) is found in Africa and has a somewhat similar progression to that of *Onchocerca.* It is spread by the **Chrysops biting fly.**

    C. *Wuchereria bancrofti* is tropical and is spread by a variety of **mosquitoes.** The **microfilariae** are **in the blood** (causing fever, chills, and eosinophilia); granulomas from **adult worms in lymphatics** lead to **elephantiasis.**

    D. *Brugia malayi* is a Far East filaria transmitted by a variety of **mosquitoes.** It produces a disease similar to *Wuchereria* infection.

IV. DRACUNCULUS. When *Dracunculus medinensis* (Guinea worm) larvae in tiny aquatic **copepods** are ingested and become mature, painful **subcutaneous lesions** (often on a foot) develop. **Adult *Dracunculus* (up to 1 meter)** may be removed by a very careful slow pull (**rolled on a stick** and eased by antiparasitic drugs) or may be removed surgically. **Filtration of drinking water through clean t-shirt material to remove the crustaceans** has nearly eradicated *Dracunculus* infection in humans in some areas.

V. ANIMAL ROUNDWORMS may infect humans, but **humans are dead-end hosts.**

    A. **Dog or cat ascarids** penetrate human skin but not the vasculature, so they "creep" around in cutaneous and subcutaneous tissues, causing **cutaneous larva migrans.**

    B. Dog and cat *Toxocara* nematodes (*T. canis* and *T. cati*) are generally asymptomatic in humans. They are associated with **pica.**

VI. TREATMENT OF NEMATODE INFECTION. Albendazole is now the drug of choice for all roundworms except *Strongyloides*.

VI
Infectious Diseases

"Paper" exam cases, such as those on the USMLE Step 1 exam, naturally are different from the real cases encountered in the practice of medicine. Paper cases generally fall into one of two categories: (1) a common disease with fairly clear presentation and either a major known causative agent (**CA**) or easily distinguished multiple CAs; or (2) an uncommon but serious disease with a distinctive presentation and CA. For example, diphtheria is a serious and distinctive disease (with a toxin), so it is more likely to be featured in a paper case than is viral meningitis, which has many viral CAs.

The following section, consisting of Chapters 35 through 43, presents infectious diseases as high-yield cases—brief case abstracts with no unnecessary details. The format is designed for both study and self-testing. For self-testing, cover each page with a piece of paper and uncover one line at a time. The question icon **QU** indicates the transition from the case information to questions related to the case; the questions are based on the most likely test material. Stop at the arrow (↙) to formulate your answers; check your answers; then move on to the next case.

35

Eye and Ear Infections

I. EYE INFECTIONS AND CONDITIONS

A. A painful swelling around an eyelash follicle ⦿ Causative agent (CA)? Name of swelling? ↙

    Staphylococcus aureus; stye (hordeolum)

B. Bilateral eyelid swelling along with muscle pain and eosinophilia ⦿ CA? ↙

    Trichinella spiralis

C. Unilateral swelling around one eye; infection may lead to enlarged flaccid heart; associated with South or Central American travel or residence ⦿ CA? Transmission? ↙

    Trypanosoma cruzi; sandfly bite

D. Conjunctivitis (red eye)

    1. First day of life; watery exudate and hyperemia ⦿ CA? ↙

        No infectious agent—silver nitrate susceptibility

    2. Neonate (1–4 days old) with hyperpurulent exudate; Gram-negative (Gr−) bacterium ⦿ CA? Seriousness? ↙

        Neisseria gonorrhoeae. It is rapidly destructive and causes irreversible damage.

    3. Neonate (3–10 days) with purulent conjunctivitis, inclusion bodies seen in cells ⦿ CA? Which serotypes? ↙

        Chlamydia trachomatis; serotypes D-K

    4. Purulent postneonatal conjunctivitis ⦿ Gram + CA? Gram − CAs? ↙

        Streptococcus pneumoniae or *Haemophilus influenzae* (formerly *H. aegyptius*)

    5. Conjunctivitis in children, with watery exudate ± sore throat; often associated with swimming ⦿ CA? Why swimming association? ↙

        Adenovirus, a naked capsid virus, so it is somewhat resistant to chlorination

E. Follicular conjunctivitis leading to inturned eyelashes, corneal scarring, and loss of vision; found in deserts of southwestern U.S., especially in Native Americans ⦿ CA? Serotypes? Disease? ↙

    Chl. trachomatis serotypes A, B, Ba, C; trachoma

F. Eye pain and ulcers from (1) wearing extended wear contacts too long or (2) being in a coma ⒬CA? ↙

Pseudomonas aeruginosa

G. Chorioretinitis in neonate or AIDS patient (sometimes lesions are described as looking like catsup and mustard) ⒬CA? ↙

Toxoplasma gondii is most common.

II. EAR INFECTIONS

A. Acute otitis media with effusion ⒬CAs?

Streptococcus pneumoniae is most common, but also nontypeable *Haemophilus influenzae* or *Moraxella catarrhalis* (Gr− diplococci), and other bacteria. Viruses include respiratory syncytial virus (RSV), adenovirus, or influenza.

B. Otitis malignant externa in diabetics ⒬CA? ↙

Pseudomonas aeruginosa

36

Respiratory Tract Infections

I. UPPER RESPIRATORY TRACT INFECTIONS AND MANIFESTATIONS

A. Exudative, erythematous pharyngitis; fever > 101°F (38.3°C), cervical lymphadenitis; rapid-antigen screen positive; backup cultures show beta-hemolytic, Gram-positive (Gr+) cocci inhibited by A disk. ⊕ Causative agent (CA)? What is in the A disk? ↙

Streptococcus pyogenes (Group A Strep); bacitracin

B. Teen or young adult with severe fatigue, pharyngitis, cervical lymphadenopathy, spleen enlargement, abnormal WBCs. Group A Strep rapid-antigen screen and backup cultures are negative. ⊕ CA? What types of WBCs are the abnormal WBCs? With what do heterophile antibodies cross-react? ↙

Epstein-Barr virus. Downey type II cells are reactive T-cells. Heterophile antibodies cross-react with animal RBCs, not with any viral antigens.

C. Pharyngitis with fever less than 101°F (38.3°C); Group A Strep rapid-antigen screen negative, backup cultures negative. ⊕ CA? Describe the virus. ↙

Adenoviruses; naked ds DNA viruses with fibers

D. Child with sore throat, fever, and gray-white papulovesicular lesions on soft palate, anterior pillars of the tonsillar fauces, uvula, and tonsil; generally without gingivitis. ⊕ CA? Disease name? Replicative intermediate? ↙

Coxsackie A; herpangina. Replicative intermediate is (−) RNA.

E. Unvaccinated child, recently arrived from former Soviet Union, presenting with sore throat with dirty pseudomembrane and heart irregularity. ⊕ CA? Disease? How does the major virulence factor work? ↙

Corynebacterium diphtheriae; diphtheria. A-B component exotoxin is produced, which ADP-ribosylates EF-2, turning off protein synthesis; mainly affected are nerve and heart cells.

F. Common cold ⊕ CA prominent in summer or fall? CA in winter or spring? ↙

Rhinovirus (summer/fall); coronavirus (winter/spring)

G. Sinus pain and inflammation ⊕ CAs? ↙

Most commonly *Streptococcus pneumoniae*; less commonly *Moraxella catarrhalis* (Gram negative and more drug resistant)

H. Paranasal swelling, hemorrhagic exudate in eyes or nose in a ketoacidotic or leukemic patient; mental lethargy ⓠ CAs? What would you expect to see in the tissues? ✘

Rhizopus or *Mucor* or *Absidia*. All three are nonseptate, extremely rapid growing, filamentous fungi with branching at nearly right angles.

I. Fever, chills, upper respiratory symptoms, severe arthralgias, and myalgias between November and March in the northern temperate zones. Leads to secondary pneumonias, particularly in the elderly. ⓠ CA? What explains major changes in the virus leading to pandemics? ✘

Influenza virus; gene reassortment (genetic shift)

J. Starts with coldlike symptoms, progresses to a repetitive cough ending in an inspiratory whoop and, often vomiting. ⓠ CA? Mechanism of the major virulence factor? ✘

Bordetella pertussis; pertussis toxin ADP-ribosylates G_i

K. Viral look-alike to pertussis ⓠ CA? ✘

Adenovirus

L. Croup; positive hemagglutination inhibition test ⓠ CA? ✘

Parainfluenza virus

M. Epiglottitis, generally in child < 3 years old; male > female; presents with drooling, needs to lean forward to breathe. ⓠ CA? What part of well baby care is child most likely missing? ✘

Haemophilus influenzae; vaccine of polyribitol capsular material linked to protein

II. BRONCHITIS AND BRONCHIOLITIS

A. Bronchiolitis in infant or child younger than 2 years old ⓠ CA? ✘

Adenovirus

B. Bronchiolitis in child 2–5 years old ⓠ CA if hemagglutinin negative? If hemagglutinin positive? ✘

Respiratory syncytial virus (hemagglutinin negative); parainfluenza virus (hemagglutinin positive)

C. Bronchitis in asthmatic patient ⓠ CAs? ✘

Most commonly viral, but also *S. pneumoniae*, *H. influenzae*, *Moraxella catarrhalis*. (USMLE exam questions would provide specifics if bacterial.)

III. PNEUMONIA (*Note:* **Age is an important predictor of the most common causative agent.** The most common CA is listed first. If you are asked to provide other CAs on the exam, you will be given specific CA characteristics.)

A. Pneumonia in nonfebrile neonate who presents with a staccato cough, no inspiratory whoop, ± conjunctivitis, and respiratory distress; x-ray pattern infiltrative, hyperinflation of lungs. ⓠ CAs? What is the infective form? ✘

Most commonly *Chlamydiae trachomatis*, which is acquired at birth but may not show clinically until 3 months. The transmitted form is the elementary body. There are many other CAs (but none as distinctive): cytomegalovirus (CMV), rubella, herpes simplex virus (HSV), *Strep. agalactiae*, and *Strep. pneumoniae*.

B. Pneumonia in child 1–3 months old. ⓠ CAs? ✍

Chlamydia trachomatis (as above), RSV or other respiratory virus, or *Bordetella* (very severe in young)

C. Pneumonia in a child 3 months to 5 years old ⓠ CAs? ✍

Generally viral (RSV or other) but also *Strep. pneumoniae, Chlamydia, Haemophilus influenzae, Mycoplasma*

D. Pneumonia in a child 5–18 years old; sore throat leading to nonproductive persistent hacking cough; no growth on blood agar, mixed flora on induced sputum. ⓠ CA? What antibiotic would *not* be effective? What is required growth factor? ✍

Mycoplasma (the most common CA in this age group; incidence decreases with increasing age). Beta-lactam antibiotics are *not* effective; sterols are growth factor.

E. In all age groups, the most common causative agent of lobar pneumonia presenting with fever and productive cough with blood-tinged sputum. ⓠ CA? What is catalase reaction of this organism? ✍

S. pneumoniae (also most common in alcoholics, people > 60 years, or smokers). It is catalase negative.

F. Pneumonia in adult with upper respiratory symptoms, diffuse infiltrates, and hypoxemia (November to March) ⓠ CA? ✍

Viral pneumonia, possibly influenza

G. Other causes of bacterial pneumonia ⓠ CAs? Distinguishing features of each? (Write out answer!) ✍

Haemophilus influenzae (Gr−, may be lobar); *Chlamydia pneumoniae* (non Gramstaining, generally mild disease); *Staphylococcus aureus* (Gr+, catalase +, may be lobar); *Legionella* spp. (acquired from air conditioning; poorly Gram staining, atypical, requires charcoal yeast extract [CYE] medium); *Chlamydia psittaci* (after exposure to sick birds or their dried excretions)

H. Pneumonia in patient who has aspirated and now has foul-smelling sputum ⓠ CA? ✍

Anaerobes

I. Pneumonia in an AIDS patient with a dry cough who is not receiving any prophylactic drugs ⓠ CA if silver staining cysts? If acid fast bacteria? If spherules? If tiny intracellular yeasts? ✍

Cysts: *Pneumocystis carinii*.

Acid-fast bacteria: *Mycobacterium tuberculosis* or M. *avium-intracellulare*.

Spherules: *Coccidioides*.

Tiny yeasts: *Histoplasma capsulatum*.

J. Pneumonia in an AIDS patient with purulent sputum ⓠ CA? ✍

S. pneumoniae

K. Pneumonia in teenage cystic fibrosis patient ⊕ CA? ↙

   Pseudomonas aeruginosa

L. Arthropod bite leading to enlarged lymph nodes, high fever, conjunctivitis, and often pneumonia; found in southeastern U.S. ⊕ CA? ↙

   Yersinia pestis

M. Pneumonia in an older male smoker and heavy drinker. Two of his bar buddies have the same acute onset of pneumonia with major headache, mental confusion, and diarrhea but no sputum. Organism does not grow on blood agar. ⊕ CA? What medium is required? ↙

   Mainly *Legionella pneumophila* and *L. micdadei*; poorly Gram staining, atypical pneumonia, CYE medium required (has cysteine and extra "iron")

N. Pneumonia with environmental associations:

   1. Contact with sick birds or dried bird excretions ⊕ CA? ↙

      Chlamydia psittaci

   2. Contact with dust enriched with bird or bat feces, in great river valleys of central U.S. ⊕ CA? ↙

      Histoplasma capsulatum

   3. Contact with desert sand of southwestern U.S. ⊕ CA? ↙

      Coccidioides immitis

37

Nervous System Infections

I. MENINGITIS

A. Viral meningitis (often called aseptic meningitis) has a tendency to be self-resolving and less acute than bacterial meningitis. ⓠ Causative agents (CAs)? ↙

Enteroviruses (like coxsackieviruses and echoviruses) as well as mumps, polio, and some of the arboviruses.

B. Purulent meningitis, rapid onset, all ages except neonates ⓠ CA? Highest number of cases in what groups? ↙

Streptococcus pneumoniae is the most common causative agent of meningitis, with highest number of cases in the very young (except neonates) and in people > 65 years of age.

C. Meningitis in neonates, particularly if there is a prolonged rupture of membranes. ⓠ Most common CA? What test could be used to identify? Other CAs? ↙

Streptococcus agalactiae (Group B) is the most common causative agent (although increased awareness is leading to a decrease in incidence of this type of meningitis). CAMP test identifies it. The second most common CA is *Escherichia coli*. Much less common is *Listeria monocytogenes*, which causes abscesses and granulomas in the fetus and a poor prognosis if it crosses the placenta. When acquired at birth, *L. monocytogenes* leads to meningitis but is much less common than *Strep. agalactiae* and *Escherichia coli*.

D. Meningitis in babies 6 months to 2 years old who are not vaccinated. ⓠ CA? Describe current vaccine. ↙

Haemophilus influenzae (Gr−) is still a problem, mostly in unvaccinated children. Vaccine is polyribitol capsule linked to protein.

E. Febrile college-age student is difficult to rouse or comatose and has cutaneous rash. ⓠ CA? What population is affected? Describe current vaccine. ↙

Neisseria meningitidis is the CA. It is epidemic and can affect any age, although there are larger numbers of cases among 1 year olds and young adults (there is a strong association with college bars). Current vaccines are used routinely in the military and consist of the Y, W-135, C, and A capsular polysaccharides. (● <u>YWCA</u> [Young <u>Women's</u> Christian Association] vaccine is used by the military [mostly young <u>men</u>].)

F. Meningitis in AIDS and immunocompromised patients ⓠCA in AIDS or immuno-compromised (except transplant) patients? CA in transplant patients? ↙

Cryptococcus neoformans (monomorphic yeast) in AIDS or most immunocompromised patients; *Listeria monocytogenes* in transplant patients

G. Meningitis in a severely neutropenic patient ⓠCA? Describe the organism. ↙

Aspergillus sp., mainly *Asp. fumigatus;* monomorphic filamentous fungus with acute branching

H. Two uncommon bacterial causes of meningitis ⓠCA if spirochetes with hooked ends? Transmission? CA if acid-fast bacilli are seen? ↙

Leptospira ("aseptic," transmitted by animal urine in water); *Mycobacterium tuberculosis*

II. BRAIN ABSCESSES

A. Aerobic, partially acid-fast, Gr+ rods and filaments on microscopy ⓠCA? ↙

Nocardia

B. Anaerobic, not acid-fast, filaments and rods seen on microscopy ⓠCA? ↙

Actinomyces

III. ENCEPHALITIS

A. Encephalitis often seen in young adults; high fatality if not treated; CSF near normal; RBCs in all four tubes of CSF. ⓠCA? Drug of choice? ↙

Herpes simplex virus (HSV) type 1; acyclovir

B. Types of mosquito-borne encephalitis ⓠWith bird reservoir? Deaths more common in elderly? Deaths more common in young? ↙

Equine encephalitis (EE); St. Louis encephalitis; California and La Crosse viruses

C. Meningoencephalitis with disturbance in smelling; associated with swimming or diving in hot waters ⓠCA? ↙

Naegleria

IV. PARESTHESIA. Paresthesia with bronze rash or nodular lesions on cool parts of body; culture negative; acid-fast bacteria in lesions ⓠCA? ↙

Mycobacterium leprae

V. VIRUSES LATENT IN NERVES

A. Virus latent in sensory nerve ganglia, with unilateral reactivation involving 1–3 dermatomes ⓠCA? ↙

Varicella-zoster virus

B. Virus latent in the trigeminal nerve ganglia ⓠCA? ↙

Herpes simplex virus 1

C. Virus latent in S-2, S-3 ⓠ CA? ↙

Herpes simplex virus 2

VI. NEUROTOXINS PRODUCED BY MICROBES

A. Patient with rigid spasm, trismus (lockjaw), severe spasms on slight noise, opisthotonus, risus sardonicus ⓠ CA? Mechanism of pathogenicity? ↙

Clostridium tetani. Its toxin blocks acetyl choline receptor.

B. Patient with flaccid paralysis ⓠ CA? Mechanism of pathogenicity? ↙

Clostridium botulinum. Toxin blocks the release of GABA and glycine.

C. Patient with dysentery and severe headache ⓠ CA? Describe. ↙

Shigella dysenteriae type I (acquired abroad). Shiga toxin has neurotoxic activities in addition to its cytotoxic and enterotoxic activities; Shigellae are invasive as well.

VII. SLOW VIRAL DISEASE

A. Progressive multifocal encephalopathy ⓠ CA? Viral family? ↙

JC virus, a polyomavirus belonging to the Papovavirus family (ds DNA with envelope)

B. Subacute sclerosing panencephalitis ⓠ CA? ↙

Measles virus

VIII. PRION DISEASE. Subacute spongiform encephalopathy ⓠ Human disease names? ↙

Creutzfeldt-Jakob disease and Kuru

38

Gastrointestinal and Hepatobiliary Disease

I. VOMITING AND DIARRHEA CAUSED BY INGESTION OF MICROBIAL TOXIN

A. Vomiting and diarrhea 1–6 hours after eating contaminated and poorly refrigerated cream pastries, ham, potato salad; no fever ⓠ Causative agent(s) (CA)? Describe toxin stability. ✔

> *Staphylococcus aureus*; the ingested enterotoxin is stable to 60°F (15°C) for 10 minutes.

B. Vomiting 1–6 hours after eating fried rice ⓠ CA? ✔

> *Bacillus cereus* producing emetic toxin

II. NONINFLAMMATORY DIARRHEA (VIRUS, NONINVASIVE BACTERIUM, OR *GIARDIA*)

A. Watery diarrhea ± vomiting after travel in developing country, but no dramatic dehydration ⓠ CA? ✔

> Enterotoxic *Escherichia coli* (ETEC)

B. Clear diarrhea with mucous flecks ± vomiting after travel in developing country; large fluid loss and rapid dehydration ⓠ CA? What is the virulence factor? ✔

> *Vibrio cholerae*. Cholera toxin is an A-B component toxin; the A component is internalized and ADP-ribosylates G_s alpha, keeping it in a persistent "on" state.

C. Infant or toddler with prolonged watery diarrhea (fall/winter/spring in temperate climate) ⓠ CA? Is it inflammatory, secretory, or malabsorptive? Describe the viral family. ✔

> Rotavirus; secretory diarrhea; naked ds RNA virus

D. Outbreak of nausea, vomiting, and nonbloody, watery diarrhea in five of six family members, 24–36 hours after attending a large church potluck. Their 9-month-old is unaffected. ⓠ CA? Why is baby unaffected? What is mode of transmission? ✔

> Norwalk agent. Baby did not eat any contaminated food. Transmission from food prepared by sick person or from shellfish from contaminated water.

E. Steatorrheic, foul-smelling diarrhea and intense abdominal cramping in patients who have camped in pristine Northern wilderness camping area and have drunk mountain stream water. ⓠ CA? Describe the pathogenic mechanism. Why does milk increase abdominal discomfort? ✔

Giardia lamblia. Attachment through the ventral sucking disk "coats" the duodenum-jejunum; large numbers ultimately cause malabsorption and a transient reduction in lactase levels

F. Voluminous watery diarrhea with crampy abdominal pain, flatulence, and weight loss; self-limiting in about 2 weeks in immunocompetent people; no effective treatment in immunocompromised patients (may involve biliary tract and may cause death); often acquired through water; acid-fast oocysts seen in intestinal brush biopsy or in diarrhea ⓆCA? ✐

Cryptosporidium parvum

G. Abdominal cramps and frankly bloody diarrhea without pus; PMNs not in excess of level in peripheral blood ⓆCA? Why are antibiotics generally contraindicated, especially in children? ✐

Escherichia coli 0157:H7 or some other enterotoxic (verotoxic) strain. There is some evidence that antibiotics may increase the risk of hemolytic uremic syndrome, particularly in children.

H. Watery diarrhea lasting 2–3 weeks in infant in developing country ⓆCA? Contrast other most likely infant diarrhea. ✐

Enteropathogenic *E. coli* (EPEC). Rotavirus is shorter and has a broader age range.

I. Explosive diarrhea with severe abdominal cramps, vomiting, and fever after ingestion of raw shellfish ⓆCA? ✐

Vibrio parahaemolyticus

III. INFLAMMATORY DIARRHEA AND DYSENTERY. Dysentery or inflammatory diarrheas result when tissue is invaded. USMLE Step 1 cases will generally include basic lab data for the organism. Fever is more prominent than in noninflammatory diarrhea, and mucus will show an excess of PMNs (over levels in peripheral blood).

A. Most common inflammatory diarrhea in U.S.; the contamination is from improper handling of raw poultry; isolate is oxidase-positive (distinguishing it from any Enterobacteriaceae); it grows at 42°C and may cause a reactive arthritis. ⓆCA? Describe O_2 intolerance or needs. ✐

Campylobacter jejuni; it is a microaerophile so it likes ~5% O_2.

B. Inflammatory diarrhea associated with poultry; oxidase-negative, G− rod, which is invasive (although the most common species rarely invades blood vessels); the major cause of osteomyelitis in sickle cell disease patients because it has a capsule. ⓆCA? Most common species? ✐

Salmonella spp. Most common in diarrhea is *S. enteritidis.*

C. Watery diarrhea progressing to abrupt onset of febrile disease with abdominal cramps, headache, tenesmus, mucoid stools with or without blood; it may be associated with daycare; stools show excess of PMNs, and organism isolated is nonlactose-fermenting, nonmotile Enterobacteriaceae with no animal reservoirs. ⓆCA? Most common species? Which is most serious and why? ✐

Shigella. In the U.S., *Shigella sonnei* is most common. Most serious is *Shigella dysenteriae* type I, which may progress to hemolytic uremic syndrome because of production of Shiga toxin.

D. Abdominal pain, fever, weight loss, generally in association with international travel, ± dysentery (blood and pus in stools) and flask-shaped intestinal lesions; extraintestinal abscesses (especially in liver) are common. ⓠCA? ↙

Entamoeba histolytica

E. Antibiotic-associated diarrhea (except amoxicillin-clavulanate, cefixime, and cefoperazone), especially if there are systemic symptoms of fever, colitis, and cramps with leukocytosis and fecal leukocytes ⓠCA? Pathogenic process? ↙

Clostridium difficile. Although many antibiotics cause diarrhea, the reduction of intestinal bacteria with the overgrowth of C. *difficile* starts with diarrhea and develops into pseudomembranous colitis (characterized by colitis with cramps, leukocytosis, or fecal leukocytes, and the ultimate development of a yellowish pseudomembrane).

IV. HEPATOBILIARY DISEASE

A. Review Table 20-2.

B. Infectious causes of cirrhosis including one parasite ⓠCA? ↙

Chronic hepatitis B, C, or B/D, but also *Schistosoma mansoni*

C. Bile duct blockage after surgery, fever, or antibiotics ⓠCA? Why does it happen? ↙

Ascaris lumbricoides. Blockage occurs because of worm size and the hypermotility under those conditions.

39

Cardiovascular Infections; Septicemias; and Blood Cell Changes in Infection

I. CARDIAC INVOLVEMENT

A. Native valve endocarditis

   1. Acute infective endocarditis ⓠ Causative agent (CA)? Why is it an acute presentation? ↙

   Staphylococcus aureus. Rapid damage is due to pore-forming alpha toxin.

   2. Subacute infective endocarditis is most likely to occur in the elderly or in those with some pre-existing heart disease.

   a. In males after urological manipulations ⓠ CA? ↙

   Enterococcus faecalis

   b. In people with pre-existing heart damage and very poor oral hygiene or with recent dental work without prophylactic antibiotics ⓠ CA? ↙

   Viridans streptococci

   3. Endocarditis in some homeless persons; no growth on blood agar ⓠ CA? ↙

   Bartonella henselae or *Bartonella quintana*

   4. Endocarditis most common in intravenous drug abusers ⓠ CA and why? What valve is involved most commonly? ↙

   Staphylococcus aureus, because of abusers' heavy skin flora of *S. aureus*; tricuspid valve. IV drug abusers have many other agents of infective endocarditis but they are less common, so they would require additional clues like a coagulase negative agent (*S. epidermidis*).

B. Endocarditis involving the prosthetic valve ⓠ CAs? ↙

   S. epidermidis, *S. aureus*, Enterobacteriaceae, *Pseudomonas*, *Aspergillus*; questions would also have to give clues about organisms here.

C. Enlarged, flabby heart leading to heart failure, resulting from infection acquired in South or Central America. ⓠ CA? Disease? Transmission? What form is found in the heart? ↙

   Trypanosoma cruzi; chronic Chagas' disease; transmitted by reduviid bug. The non-flagellated amastigotes are present in the heart muscle.

D. Pericarditis ⓠCAs? ✎

Usually viral, most commonly the Coxsackie or other enteroviruses

E. Myocarditis ⓠCAs? ✎

Also most commonly the Coxsackie or other enteroviruses, but also seen in Lyme disease

II. SEPTICEMIAS AND SHOCK. Many different infections disseminate via the bloodstream causing systemic febrile symptoms and septic shock. For example, endotoxin (Gr−), *Staphylococcus aureus* TSST-1, *Streptococcus pyogenes* SPE-A, and peptidoglycan-teichoic acid fragments of Gr+ organisms such as *Streptococcus pneumoniae* may all be causative factors. Paper cases will have to give you additional information. Most of the rickettsial diseases like Rocky Mountain spotted fever (RMSF) that cause systemic febrile disease will mention capillary and small vessel endothelial damage (and thrombus), rash, and will generally also give vector clues (e.g., *Dermacentor* ticks for RMSF). A paper case about brucellosis will include exposure to infected animals.

III. CHANGES IN BLOOD COUNTS SEEN WITH INFECTION

A. Anemias

1. Pernicious megaloblastic anemia with history of fish ingestion ⓠCA? Disease process? ✎

Diphyllobothrium latum (fish tapeworm in cool lake regions), attached high in the small intestine, competes for B_{12}, producing the anemia.

2. Microcytic hypochromic anemia ⓠCAs? Disease process? ✎

Hookworms (*Necator* or *Ancylostoma*) or *Trichuris*. Blood loss is due to intestinal attachment of a large number of worms.

3. Paroxysmal febrile disease (high fever with chills, rigors, sweats, and headache) that may become cyclic; reduced hematocrit and hemoglobin ⓠCA? Disease? ✎

Plasmodium spp.; malaria

B. Broad generalizations about white cell changes in infection

1. Lymphocytosis with severe hacking cough, generally without fever ⓠCA? ✎

Bordetella pertussis

2. Eosinophilia ⓠWhen does it occur? ✎

During worm migration or in allergic reactions

3. Mononuclear cell increase ⓠCA? ✎

Intracellular organisms like viruses, *Listeria*, or *Toxoplasma*

4. PMN increases ⓠCA? ✎

Usually extracellular bacteria

5. CD4+ cell decline to below $200/mm^3$ ⓠ ✎

AIDS

40

Bone or Joint Infections

I. ARTHRITIS

A. Polyarticular arthritis, sometimes migratory, in a 15- to 40-year-old female

1. With petechiae ⓠ Causative agent (CA)? ✔

Neisseria gonorrhoeae

2. Intermittent with preceding bullet rash and headache or history of tick bite ⓠ Disease? CA? ✔

Lyme disease; *Borrelia burgdorferi*

B. Nongonococcal infective arthritis, usually monoarticular ⓠ CA? Who is most commonly affected? ✔

Staphylococcus aureus is most common, especially in individuals with rheumatoid arthritis.

C. Arthritis with artificial joints involved ⓠ CA? ✔

Staphylococcus epidermidis or *S. aureus*

II. OSTEOMYELITIS

A. Osteomyelitis with no co-morbidity (including no trauma) ⓠ CA? CA when seen in neonates? ✔

Staphylococcus aureus; in neonates, *S. aureus*, *S. agalactiae*, and Enterobacteriaceae

B. Osteomyelitis in sickle cell disease patients ⓠ CA? What virulence factor? ✔

Salmonella (It has a capsule; *S. aureus* rarely does.) SSD patients have an extremely high rate of osteomyelitis, with more than 80% of cases caused by *Salmonella* spp.

C. Osteomyelitis after a foot wound ⓠ CAs? ✔

Pseudomonas aeruginosa, *S. aureus*

D. Osteomyelitis involving prosthetic joints ⓠ CAs? ✔

S. aureus, *S. epidermidis*

E. Osteomyelitis in intravenous drug abusers ⓠ CAs? ✔

S. aureus, *Pseudomonas aeruginosa*

41

Genitourinary Tract Infections

I. CYSTITIS

A. In all people (even young sexually active women), most common cause of cystitis ⓠⓤ Causative agent (CA)? ✘

Escherichia coli

B. In adolescent women who are newly sexually active, second most common cause of cystitis ⓠⓤ CA? What rapid diagnostic lab test would be negative? ✘

Staphylococcus saprophyticus. Nitrite test is negative.

II. BLOOD IN URINE. Symptom of routine bacterial cystitis, but when found in a patient traveling or living in a place like rural Africa ⓠⓤ CA? Disease? Route of acquisition? ✘

Schistosoma hematobium; schistosomiasis; acquired through water/skin contact

III. REPRODUCTIVE TRACT INFECTIONS

A. Vesicular genital lesions that ulcerate and recur, with significant nerve pain prior to outbreaks ⓠⓤ CA? Where latent? ✘

Herpes simplex virus 2; latent in S-2, S-3

B. Genital warts ⓠⓤ CA? Most common serotypes? ✘

Human papilloma virus; 6 and 11

C. In prepubescent girls, urethritis or vaginitis; in postpubescent females, cervicitis, endometriosis, PID, or perihepatitis; in males, epididymitis; in both sexes, possible Reiter syndrome (urethritis, iridocyclitis, and arthritis, sometimes recurring). Culture is negative on any bacteriologic medium. Diagnosis by genetic probe or tissue culture. ⓠⓤ CA? Why reinfection? ✘

Chlamydia trachomatis. Reinfection is common because of multiple serotypes (D-K).

D. In females, asymptomatic condition or urethritis, endocervicitis, or PID; in males, most commonly urethritis. Gram-negative diplococcus. ⓠⓤ CA? Current test for diagnosis? Culture medium and conditions? ✘

Neisseria gonorrhoeae; genetic probe tests for diagnosis; culture on Thayer-Martin agar in high CO_2

E. Most commonly seen now in female IV drug abusers or sex workers, or in promiscuous male homosexuals. Painless, indurated genital lesions that ulcerate with a fairly clean (not ragged) border. These primary chancres may heal spontaneously but disease (without treatment) may progress to mucocutaneous lesions on all body surfaces, including palms and soles. Skin lesions are maculopapular; mucous membranes are often grayish, hypertrophic, papular, and more likely to transmit infection than the drier skin lesions. There are also systemic signs such as fever, lymphadenopathy, malaise, and enlarged spleen. Gram stain of any lesion will be negative (meaning no notable pathogen seen, as opposed to "Gram-negative bacteria seen"). ⓠ CA? Disease? How is diagnosis reached? ↙

Treponema pallidum; syphilis; serodiagnosis with dark-field or fluorescent microscopy of chancre exudate or mucous membrane secondary lesions; not cultured in clinical labs.

F. Painful, soft chancre; slow to heal, which increases risk of transmission of AIDS. ⓠ CA? Describe organism. ↙

Haemophilus ducreyi (ⓜ You do cry with ducreyi); Gram-negative rod

G. In females, asymptomatic or irritating vaginitis with malodorous, thin yellowish green discharge (numerous PMNs); discharge pH 5–6 and may give a positive amine test ("whiff" test) when mixed with KOH; vagina congested or with punctate hemorrhages. In males, urethritis ⓠ CA? ↙

Trichomonas vaginalis

H. Pruritic, painful vulvovaginitis with normal pH (4–4.5) and pseudohyphae seen on microscopy ⓠ CA? ↙

Candida albicans

I. Malodorous vaginal discharge; usually worse with intercourse because ejaculate is basic; usually nonpainful intercourse. Discharge is homogeneous and somewhat adherent, and generally gives a positive amine test. Microscopy shows an increased number of coccobacilli. "Clue" cells (epithelial cells covered with bacteria) are present. ⓠ CA? Disease? ↙

Gardnerella vaginalis at higher levels than normal; bacterial vaginosis

42

Cancers Associated with Infections

I. CANCERS ASSOCIATED WITH VIRUSES

A. Cervical cancer ⓠ Associated agent (AA)? Mechanism of carcinogenesis? How transferred? Associated with what other carcinoma? ↙

Human papilloma virus (HPV) strains 16 and 18 carry genes that produce early proteins which interfere with normal tumor suppressor gene function. E6 interferes with p53 and E7 with Rb (p110). These are sexually transferred and also associated with penile carcinoma.

B. Burkitt's lymphoma ⓠ AAs? ↙

Epstein Barr virus (EBV) in malarious regions. In a person co-infected with EBV and *Plasmodium*, chromosomal translocation may occur, resulting in lymphoma.

C. Liver carcinoma ⓠ AAs and type of infection? ↙

Hepatitis B or C chronic infections

D. Human T-cell leukemias or lymphomas ⓠ AA? ↙

Human T-cell leukemia virus (HTLV)

II. CANCERS ASSOCIATED WITH PARASITES

A. Bladder carcinoma ⓠ AA? ↙

Schistosoma haematobium chronic infection

B. *Plasmodium* ⓠ Carcinoma association? ↙

Burkitt's lymphoma; as above in I B

43

Skin and Subcutaneous Infections; Rashes

I. SKIN AND SUBCUTANEOUS INFECTIONS

A. Surgical wounds or carbuncles (boils) or furuncles (multiple ulcerating boils) ⓠ Causative agent (CA)? ↙

   Staphylococcus aureus

B. Swollen jaw following dental trauma or work; may ulcerate to the surface with the presence of "sulfur" granules in the exudate. ⓠ CA? Description of causative agent? What are the granules? ↙

   CA: *Actinomyces israelii*, a bacterium! It is a Gr+ anaerobe that is not acid-fast. Granules are microcolonies.

C. Dermatitis along tight areas of swimsuit after swimming ⓠ Name of ailment? CA? ↙

   Swimmer's itch from infection with "nonhuman" schistosomes

D. Itchy skin lesions spreading out from the periphery; margins usually erythematous; appear anywhere on body; KOH[1] shows hyphae and arthroconidia. ⓠ Type of infection? Specific causative agents and tissues each agent infects? ↙

   Dermatophyte infection (tinea):
   - *Microsporum* invades hair and skin.
   - *Trichophyton* invades hair, nails, and skin.
   - *Epidermophyton* invades skin and nails.

E. Impetigo caused by a Gram-positive coccus positive for both catalase and coagulase. ⓠ CA? Typical clinical appearance? ↙

   Staphylococcus aureus; may have bullae (or be described as bullous)

F. Swollen subcutaneous lesion (or chain of lesions) resulting from trauma involving plant materials such as plum tree, rose or other thorny plant, or floral wire; occupational hazard of greenhouse and plant nursery workers and gardeners ⓠ Disease? CA? Description of CA in environment *vs* in humans? ↙

   Disease: Sporotrichosis. *Sporothrix schenckii*, the CA, is a dimorphic fungus that is filamentous in the environment; in human tissues it forms sparse cigar-shaped and oval yeasts.

---

[1]KOH = microscopic examination of potassium hydroxide–mounted skin scales

G. A primary concern with deep puncture wounds or any complex dirty wound ⓠ CA? Most common infectious form? Mechanism of pathogenicity? ↙

Clostridium tetani; spores and vegetative cells; neurotoxin production causes rigid paralysis.

H. Cellulitis caused by nail through bottom of tennis shoe ⓠ CA? Where is organism coming from? ↙

Pseudomonas aeruginosa is the most common CA. The organism comes from the inside of the tennis shoe (rubber sole "cleans up" outside dirt on nail).

I. Wound contaminated with fecal material or soil, leading to the production of gas trapped in tissues and gangrene. ⓠ CA? Major toxin? ↙

Clostridium perfringens; alpha toxin, a lecithinase

J. Necrotizing fasciitis ⓠ CA? ↙

Streptococcus pyogenes

K. Superficial peeling of large areas of skin ⓠ CA? Disease? ↙

Staphylococcus aureus; scalded skin syndrome due to exfoliatins

L. Diaper rash with sharply demarcated red to normal skin with a few punctate red dots on the normal skin ⓠ CA? What would be seen on microscopy? ↙

Candida spp.; *pseudohyphae, hyphae and yeasts* on microscopy

M. Impetigo caused by a catalase-negative organism, usually described as a honey-crusted lesion ⓠ CA? ↙

Streptococcus pyogenes

N. Burned tissue with blue-green pus and odd, sweet, grapelike odor ⓠ CA? ↙

Pseudomonas aeruginosa

O. Dermatitis with fairly intense itching which develops after walking barefoot on a tropical beach ⓠ Most likely CA? Disease? Other CAs? ↙

CA: Dog ascarids that infect humans. Disease: cutaneous larva migrans. Other causes include repeated hookworm (*Necator* or *Ancylostoma*) or *Strongyloides* infections from walking barefoot on soil.

P. Pink umbilicate warts with central debris ⓠ CA? Pathology clue? Viral family? ↙

CA: Molluscum contagiosum virus. Clue: molluscum bodies in cell cytoplasm. Viral family: Poxviridae.

Q. Patient working with animal, animal skins, or wool develops a red tumorlike lesion with central necrosis and a raised red margin. ⓠ CA? Disease? Unique virulence factors? ↙

CA: *Bacillus anthracis.* Disease: anthrax. Virulence factors: polypeptide capsule and two toxins (LF, EF) that share a B component (protective antigen, or PA).

II. RASHES. In general, vesicular rashes are more often viral than bacterial; *Staphylococcus* may cause vesicles or bullae.

A. Vesiculate rash starts in hair and behind ears and spreads downward, with major concentration on trunk and sparse distribution on limbs. The rash is asynchronous (the initially vesicular lesion quickly ulcerates and crusts over, and there are progressive new crops of lesions). Fever ranges up to 103°F (39.4°C) for a few days after the rash starts. ⓠ CA? Disease ✔

Varicella zoster virus; chickenpox

B. Seasonal infection (from deep winter to early spring) beginning with cough, coryza, and conjunctivitis, with fever ranging from 101° to 103°F (38° to 39.4°C) prior to the onset of rash. (White oral buccal lesions with a red base appear on days 3 to 6 but often are not noted.) Blotchy red rash starts on face and spreads downward, becoming confluent on face and upper trunk while remaining discrete on lower extremities ⓠ Disease (common and formal names)? CA? ✔

Measles (rubeola); measles virus

C. Painful outbreak of vesiculate lesions along 1 to 3 dermatomes ⓠ CA? Disease? ✔

Varicella zoster virus; shingles

D. Symptoms include sore throat, often with yellowish tonsillar exudate; strawberry tongue; fever; and sparse, fine, "sandpaper" rash that blanches on pressure and usually starts on cheeks, sparing circumoral area, with increased density at neck, axillae, and groin ⓠ Disease? CA? Virulence factor? ✔

Disease: scarlet fever. CA: *Streptococcus pyogenes*. Virulence factor: SPE-A, B, or C is the erythrogenic toxin.

E. Teen to young adult with exudative sore throat, fever, lymphadenopathy, and fatigue; when given ampicillin, develops major rash with no change in throat ⓠ CA? Describe CA. ✔

Epstein Barr virus; enveloped DNA virus (icosahedral)

F. Febrile child, not very sick, with red cheeks and thin lacy rash on body; condition usually seen in late spring ⓠ CA? Disease? ✔

Parvovirus B19; fifth disease ("slapped cheek fever")

G. Child 5 months to 3 years with high fever for 3 days; maculopapular facial rash appears after fever abates ⓠ CA? Disease? ✔

Human herpesvirus 6; exanthem subitum (roseola infantum)

H. Acute onset of illness: healthy person suddenly becomes very ill, with mental confusion and petechiae very quickly developing into purpura and shock ⓠ CA? disease? ✔

Neisseria meningitidis causing meningococcemia and meningitis

VII
Comparative Microbiology

This section is a "review of the review," providing you with horizontal comparisons of microbes, features, virulence factors, and so on. As in the previous section, you can test yourself. Use a cover sheet, reading down line by line until you hit a list heading. Then, on a separate sheet of paper, using abbreviations, quickly write your own list. Compare it to the one given, then add the ones you missed to your list. This, along with the flow charts in Chapter 7, makes a good last-minute review. If you just want to read through these lists, be sure to make a separate list of the items you don't know for later study.

44

High-Yield Microbial Clues and Comparisons

I. VIRULENCE FACTORS AND FEATURES IMPORTANT IN DISEASE

A. Surface adherence and colonization

1. Gram-positive teichoic acids

2. M fimbriae of *Streptococcus pyogenes*

3. Gram-negative pili

4. IgA proteases: *Streptococcus pneumoniae*, *Neisseria* spp., *Haemophilus influenzae*

5. Biofilms
   a. *Staphylococcus epidermidis* biofilms adhere to artificial body parts and catheters.
   b. *Streptococcus mutans* biofilms cause dental plaque.

B. Antiphagocytic structures

1. **All capsules.** Capsules are the most important antiphagocytic structures. ● Some Killers Have Pretty Nice Capsules:
   a. <u>S</u>treptococcus pneumoniae
   b. <u>K</u>lebsiella pneumoniae and K1 strains of *Escherichia coli*
   c. <u>H</u>aemophilus influenzae
   d. <u>P</u>seudomonas aeruginosa
   e. <u>N</u>eisseria meningitidis
   f. <u>C</u>ryptococcus neoformans (yeast)

2. **Pili** of *Neisseria gonorrhoeae*

3. **M protein** of *Streptococcus pyogenes*

4. The **A protein** of *Staphylococcus aureus*

C. Toxins

1. **Toxins with ADP-ribosyl transferase** activity are important in disease. **Table 44-1** lists high-yield examples.

2. **Heat stability of bacterial toxins**
   a. **Toxins that are heat stable at boiling point of water, 100°C (212°F):** endotoxins
   b. **Toxins that are heat stable at 60°C (140°F) for 10 minutes**
      (1) *Staphylococcus aureus* enterotoxin
      (2) Stable toxin (ST) of *Escherichia coli*
      (3) *Yersinia enterocolitica* toxin
   c. **Toxins denatured by moderate heat:** all the rest of the bacterial toxins

Table 44-1

Toxins with ADP-Ribosyl Transferase and Resulting Conditions

Toxin	ADP-ribosylates	Result
Cholera toxin	G_s alpha protein of small intestinal cells	Stimulates G_s, increase in cAMP Massive fluid loss (diarrhea)
***E. coli* heat-labile toxin (LT)**	G_s protein of small intestinal cells	Stimulates G_s, increase in cAMP Fluid loss (diarrhea)
Pertussis toxin	G_i (inhibits the negative regulator of adenylate cyclase)	Inhibits G_i Increase in cAMP, lymphocytosis, increased insulin secretion
Diphtheria toxin	EF-2	Shuts down protein synthesis
***Pseudomonas aeruginosa* exotoxin A**	EF-2	Shuts down protein synthesis

3. Toxins that cause membrane damage: *Clostridium perfringens* alpha toxin (a lecithinase), *Staphylococcus aureus* alpha toxin (a pore-forming toxin)

4. Other toxins: For review, see toxins in Table 4-1, Chapter 4.

D. Other virulence factors

1. Coagulase: *Staphylococcus aureus* and *Yersinia pestis*

2. Urease: *Cryptococcus neoformans*, *Nocardia*, *Helicobacter pylori*, *Proteus*, and *Ureaplasma* (The last two, especially *Proteus*, increase urine pH in urinary tract infections, causing kidney stones.)

3. Hyaluronidase: Group A streptococci and *Staphylococcus aureus*

II. IDENTIFIERS OF MICROORGANISMS

A. Stain reactions

1. Non-Gram staining or poorly seen on Gram stain
   a. Mycoplasmas, *Ureaplasma*; no cell wall
   b. *Chlamydia*, *Rickettsia*; too small
   c. Spirochetes (*Treponema*, *Borrelia*, *Leptospira*); too thin
   d. *Legionella*; Gram-negative stain seen only if counterstain time is increased

2. Acid fast
   a. Mycobacterium
   b. *Nocardia* (partially)
   c. *Legionella micdadei*
   d. *Cryptosporidium* oocysts
   e. *Isospora* oocysts

3. Silver staining
   a. Fungi
   b. *Legionella*

4. Periodic acid-Schiff: Fungi stain red.

5. Calcofluor white: Fungi fluoresce blue-white on black.

6. **India Ink wet mount:** *Cryptococcus* shows colorless cells with halos (capsular material) on black; test misses 50%.

B. **Size comparisons** of microbes. See Chapter 1, Figure 1-1, for proportional drawings of major groups of microorganisms.

C. **Special culture limitations**

1. **Intracellular pathogens:** require tissue culture; cannot be grown on inert media or cannot be grown in vitro

    a. **Obligate intracellular:** all viruses, *Chlamydia*, all Rickettsias except *Bartonella* (*Rochalimaea*), *Mycobacterium leprae*, Plasmodia, *Toxoplasma*

    b. **Facultative intracellular:** *Listeria*, all Mycobacteria, *Histoplasma*, *Brucella*

2. **Non-intracellular pathogens that cannot yet be routinely cultured:** *T. pallidum*, *Pneumocystis*

D. **Endospore formers** (Gram-positive, dipicolinic acid in core): *Bacillus*, *Clostridium*

E. **Anaerobes.** Don't worry about obligate vs. aerotolerant for the USMLE Step 1 exam. 🅜 The ABCs of anaerobiosis = Actinomyces, Bacteroides, Clostridium

F. **Microaerophilic organisms:** *Campylobacter* grows at 42°C (107.6°F), *Helicobacter* at 37°C (98.6°F).

G. **Obligate aerobes:** *Mycobacterium tuberculosis*, *Pseudomonas*

H. **Media clues and growth factors** are listed in **Table 44-2.** Quiz yourself by covering one side of the table at a time.

I. **Specific inhibitors**

1. Bacitracin ("A" disk used by labs) inhibits *Streptococcus pyogenes* (Group A).

2. Optochin ("P" disk used by labs) inhibits (and bile lyses) Pneumococcus.

J. The following are the **most likely to be pictured or physically described on the USMLE Step 1 exam:**

1. **Mycobacterium:** thin red rods on acid-fast stain (aerobic)

Table 44-2
Media Clues or Growth Factors and Organisms for Which They Are Used

Media Clue or Growth Factor	Used for Which Organism(s)?
Charcoal yeast extract agar	*Legionella*
Cholesterol	Mycoplasmas and Ureaplasmas
Salt tolerant	*Staphylococcus aureus, Enterococcus faecalis, Streptococcus bovis, Vibrio parahaemolyticus, V. vulnificus*
X and V factors	(Hematin and NADH) *Haemophilus influenzae*
Chocolate agar	*Haemophilus* and *Neisseria*
Thayer-Martin (chocolate with antibiotics)	*Neisseria*
Regan-Lowe	*Bordetella pertussis*
Lowenstein-Jensen	Mycobacteria (now automated broth systems)

2. A Gram-positive organism: intense blue to purple (tissues pale red)

3. A Gram-negative organism: pink to clear red

4. Adenovirus: icosahedral, projecting fibers. See Table 21-1, DNA Viruses.

5. *Giardia:* flagellated pyriform protozoan with a sucking disk

6. *Entamoeba histolytica:* amoeba with "wagon-wheel" nucleus and ingested RBCs

7. Dimorphic fungi: in body = yeast or yeastlike; at lower temps (cold) = mold
   a. *Blastomyces dermatitidis:* broad-based budding yeast or hyphae; possible association with wood
   b. *Coccidioides immitis:* hyphae and arthroconidia in southwestern U.S. sand; in lungs, arthroconidia develop into spherules
   c. *Histoplasma capsulatum:* hyphae with tuberculate macroconidia and microconidia in soil enriched with bird or bat feces; in tissue, facultative intracellular fungus seen as tiny oval budding yeasts
   d. *Sporothrix schenckii:* filamentous hyphae (rosettes or sleeves of conidia) on plant material; in tissue, develops into oval to cigar-shaped yeasts

III. HIGH-YIELD TRANSMISSION DATA. Table 44-3 lists important diseases and their causative agents, reservoirs, and modes of transmission. Although fecal organisms may be transmitted by oral sex, or from exposed feces by flies, the usual route is from fingers to food, or fingers to fomites as in daycare situations (a major route for fecal–oral transmission).

Table 44-3

High-Yield Guide to Diseases and their Causative Agents, Reservoirs, and Modes of Transmission

Disease	Causative Agent	Reservoir	Mode of Transmission
All STDs	*T. pallidum* *N. gonorrhoeae* *Chlamydia* HPV HSV-2, etc.	Humans only	Sexual, birth, or other direct contact; *T. pallidum* crosses the placenta
Typhoid	*Salmonella typhi*	Humans only	Fecal–oral
Leprosy	*Mycobacterium leprae*	Humans (also armadillos, man-gabey monkeys)	Respiratory droplets and direct contact
Cryptococcal pneumonia (symptomatic)	*Cryptococcus neoformans*	Pigeons	Inhalation (bridge painters, pigeon breeders)
African sleeping sickness	*Trypanosoma brucei*	Humans	Tsetse flies
Histoplasmosis	*Histoplasma capsulatum*	Soil; bird or bat feces in great river valleys in U.S.	Inhalation
Infectious hepatitis	Hepatitis A virus	Humans, water, oysters	Fecal–oral or food-borne
Bloody diarrheas	*Campylobacter* *E. coli* 0157:H7	Domestic animals Cattle	Undercooked chicken Undercooked hamburger
Salmonellosis	*Salmonella enteritidis*	Chicken, eggs	Undercooked chicken

(cont.)

Disease	Causative Agent	Reservoir	Mode of Transmission
Chagas' disease	*Trypanosoma cruzi*	Domestic animals and pets alternating with reduviid bugs	Reduviid bugs (cone or kissing bugs)
Valley fever	*Coccidioides immitis*	Desert sand of southwestern U.S	Dust (with arthroconidia) inhalation
Malaria	*Plasmodium* species	Mammals alternating with *Anopheles* mosquitoes	Mosquito bite
Leishmaniasis (all types)	*Leishmania* species	Sandflies	Sandfly bite
Lyme disease	*Borrelia burgdorferi*	Deer, deer mice, *Ixodes* ticks	*Ixodes* tick bite (nymph or adult)
Leptospirosis	*Leptospira interrogans*	Rats, cattle	Animal urine in recreational waters, or sewers
Toxoplasmosis	*Toxoplasma gondii*	Cats and all other animals including humans	Raw meat, cat feces; crosses placenta, reactivates in immunocompromised patients
Rocky Mountain spotted fever	*Rickettsia rickettsii*	Dogs and ticks	Dermacentor ticks
Legionnaire's disease	*Legionella* species	Water and amoebas	Air conditioning
Viral diarrheas	Rotavirus in infants, Norwalk virus in older persons	Humans May also be shellfish for Norwalk virus	Fecal–oral
Gray, greasy diarrhea	*Giardia lamblia*	Humans and beavers	Water, fecal–oral
Schistosomiasis	*Schistosoma* species	Snails always are one host	Water contact
Plague	*Yersinia pestis*	Small wild animals in southwestern U.S. deserts	Flea bite, or respiratory droplets
Tuberculosis	*Mycobacterium tuberculosis*	Humans	Respiratory droplets or droplet nuclei

VIII
High-Yield Case Set-ups

This section of high-yield case set-ups and related questions is designed to be used as a self-test to let you know whether you need more review. Each of the 22 items consists of a high-yield case scenario, followed by questions about the case; answers to the questions then follow. Only critical clues are given in each case. Item #4 includes case modifications that require you to select a different causative agent (CA).

Directions: Use a cover sheet to read down the page one line at a time. A question icon (⊕) separates the case information in each item from the questions about the case. Stop when you see the arrow (↙) and answer the questions, then move your cover sheet down to check your answers before moving on to the next item.

A note about causative agents: The clinical vignette questions on the USMLE Step 1 exam often do not ask for the causative agent, but **you must know the causative agent in order to answer basic science questions** about the disease or the causative agent. For this reason, every case in this appendix asks you to identify the causative agent.

A note about the use of "and" vs. "or": This self-test, like the USMLE Step 1 exam, uses the words "and" and "or" in the Boolean sense—that is, the word "or" between clues means that *any one* of these clues will affect your answer, whereas the word "and" means *all* clues apply.

45

High-Yield Case Set-Ups

1. Lobar pneumonia in an alcoholic (or elderly) patient ⓠ CA? Chemistry and function of major virulence factor? Sputum? Lab ID of CA? ↙

   CA: *Streptococcus pneumoniae* (by far the most common causative agent in alcoholics and elderly!). **Major virulence factor:** The polysaccharide capsule reduces complement activation and phagocytic engulfment. **Sputum:** Blood tinged or rusty but not foul-smelling. **Lab ID:** CA is alpha-hemolytic, inhibited by optochin (P disk), and lysed by bile (bile activates *Strep. pneumoniae* autolysins).

2. Lobar pneumonia with deep red (currant jelly) sputum *or* Gram-negative CA. ⓠ CA? What patients are most likely to have it? Associated symptom that makes treatment difficult? ↙

   CA: *Klebsiella pneumoniae.* **Likely patients:** Alcoholics and patients with COPD. **Associated symptom:** This type of pneumonia is very serious because of the high frequency of abscesses, but it is not as common as pneumonia caused by *S. pneumoniae.*

3. Pneumonia in an alcoholic with or without vomiting and passing out, *or* with foul-smelling sputum; with or without pulmonary abscesses, sometimes with visible fluid level. ⓠ CA? Where are they from? ↙

   Mixed anaerobes from aspiration of oral/pharyngeal normal flora and vomitus

4. Meningitis in neonate born after long delivery with early rupture of amniotic sac. ⓠ Most common CA? What factor increases risk? ↙

   Streptococcus agalactiae (Group B *Streptococcus*) is most common CA; major risk is prolonged membrane rupture.

   a. **Modification #1:** Meningitis occurs in neonate and CA is Gram-negative. ⓠ CA? ↙

      Escherichia coli

   b. **Modification #2:** Meningitis occurs in neonate and CA is Gram-positive rod. ⓠ CA? What other patient population is sensitive to this organism? ↙

      Listeria monocytogenes; more likely to cause meningitis in transplant patients

5. Foot swelling and redness as a result of stepping on nail which penetrates tennis shoe. ⓠ CA? What other diseases does this CA cause in other patient populations? ↙

   Pseudomonas aeruginosa. Also causes pneumonia in cystic fibrosis or severely neutropenic patients; cellulitis in burn patients; folliculitis in hot tub users; malignant otitis media in diabetics; eye ulcers in coma patients or patients using extended wear contacts

6. Knee joint pain and swelling, and skin petechiae with or without low-grade fever in a sexually active young woman ⓠ CA? Disease? What is immunity or reinfection potential following treatment? How is diagnosis made? If cultured, what medium? ↙

> **CA:** *Neisseria gonorrhoeae*. **Disease:** Arthritis from disseminated and untreated gonorrhea. **Reinfection:** Common antigenic variation of pili and outer membrane proteins results in high risk of reinfection of a person with multiple sexual partners who does not use barrier protection. **Diagnosis and culture medium:** Gonorrhea diagnosis is made with use of genetic probes. *N. gonorrhoeae* is cultured on Thayer-Martin since it will not grow well on blood agar.

7. Patient (frequently child) has acute pharyngitis with yellowish exudate, regional lymphadenopathy, often high fever; beta-hemolytic organism inhibited by bacitracin ⓠ CA? Potential suppurative sequelae if untreated? Potential non-suppurative sequelae? ↙

> **CA:** *Streptococcus pyogenes*. **Suppurative sequelae:** otitis media, sinusitis, abscesses. **Non-suppurative sequelae:** rheumatic fever (polyarthritis of large joints, carditis, erythema nodosum and marginatum, chorea) or acute glomerulonephritis

8. Vietnamese person escaped on a boat and spent 4 years in a Pacific refugee camp before coming to U.S.; now suffers from back pain, weight loss, and night sweats; X-ray film shows vertebral destruction. ⓠ CA and description? Growth medium? ↙

> *Mycobacterium tuberculosis* is an acid-fast bacterium requiring a high lipid medium to grow (Lowenstein-Jensen medium), although it is now also grown in Middlebrook broth with radioactive palmitic acid in special machines.

9. Febrile young person with rapid onset of stiff neck, mental confusion, and skin petechiae ⓠ CA? What surface component enables CA to *reach* the blood–brain barrier (BBB)? What enables it to *cross* the BBB? Which serotype is least immunogenic? Is it contagious? ↙

> **CA:** *Neisseria meningitidis* most likely. **Surface components:** Polysaccharide capsule protects the bacterium and enables it to reach the BBB. Endotoxin in the outer membrane causes inflammation that facilitates invasion of the CNS. **Least immunogenic serotype:** B capsule—composed of sialic acid, so it is not immunogenic. **Contagiousness:** It is an epidemic disease, although many more are colonized than develop disease.

10. Severely neutropenic patient with respiratory distress; bronchioalveolar lavage fluids show septate hyphal elements (filaments) with generally acute, dichotomous branching. ⓠ CA? ↙

> *Aspergillus fumigatus*; this is a *monomorphic* filamentous fungus.

11. Immigrant from lower socioeconomic class of South or Central America presents with fatigue and an enlarged heart; biopsy shows amastigotes. ⓠ CA? Disease? How acquired? How does it affect adults? What country is most affected? Why is it a concern in the U.S.? ↙

> **CA:** *Trypanosoma cruzi*. **Disease:** trypanosomiasis (Chagas' disease). **Acquired:** in poorer housing from bites of reduviid bugs (cone or kissing bugs). **In adults:** infections often chronic and lead to heart failure. **Countries:** It is a major cause of death in Brazil, and is a transfusion concern in U.S.

12. Patient presents with bone pain and tender, inflamed tissues over the painful area; no history of trauma; no underlying disease; patient not a neonate. ⓠ CA? Type of organism? Reactions to coagulase and catalase? ↙

> **CA:** *Staphylococcus aureus*, a Gram-positive coccus. **Reactions:** coagulase +, catalase +

13. Osteomyelitis in sickle-cell disease patient ⑩ CA? Why are these patients susceptible? ↙

   Salmonella enteritidis. Sickle-cell disease patients (who are asplenic from repeated infarcts and also may have a defect in complement) do not control encapsulated organisms well, so they have a very high rate of osteomyelitis. (*S. aureus* is rarely encapsulated.)

14. Profuse watery diarrhea leading to rapid and severe dehydration. ⑩ CA? Pathogenesis? Management? ↙

   Vibrio cholerae. Toxin is ADP-ribosyl transferase of G-binding protein causing increase in cAMP. High risk of hypovolemic shock unless treated with electrolytes and fluid replacement. Antibiotics reduce spread.

15. Adoptee from former Soviet Union has pharyngitis with pseudomembrane formation. ⑩ CA? Other organs likely to be involved? Pathogenesis? Definitive test? Culture medium or other distinctive clues likely to be mentioned? Prevention (type of vaccine)? ↙

   CA: *Corynebacterium diphtheriae.* **Other organs:** heart (myocarditis/heart failure) and nervous system (recurrent laryngeal palsy). **Pathogenesis:** circulating exotoxin inhibits protein synthesis through ADP ribosylation of EF-2. **Definitive test:** Elek test (agar immunodiffusion to identify toxin production). **Culture medium:** Loeffler's coagulated serum medium and tellurite-containing medium are distinctive. **Vaccine:** toxoid.

16. Woman with cervical intraepithelial neoplasia ⑩ CA and serotypes? Pathogenic mechanism? ↙

   Human papilloma virus 16 or 18. Early proteins interfere with tumor suppressor gene activity—E6 interferes with p53; E7, with p110 (Rb).

17. Wilderness camper who drank mountain stream water presents with abdominal pain and grey steatorrheic stools. ⑩ CA? How does it cause diarrhea? ↙

   Giardia lamblia fastens to duodenal and jejunal lining by ventral sucking disk, blocking absorption.

18. Hospitalized patient with enterococcal septicemia, being treated with clindamycin, develops diarrhea on the fifth day. ⑩ CA? Appropriate tests? Pathogenesis? ↙

   CA: *Clostridium difficile.* **Tests:** Do not order ova and parasites; test for presence of *C. difficile* toxins A and B. **Pathogenesis:** through exotoxin production. Toxin A is an enterotoxin and granulocyte attractant, causing mucosal damage and water and electrolyte loss. Toxin B is cytotoxin.

19. College student camping through tropical developing country develops watery (nonbloody) diarrhea. ⑩ Most likely CA if self-resolving after a couple of days of saltines and 7-Up? Pathogenesis? ↙

   Enterotoxic *E. coli.* Production of two possible exotoxins: LT ADP-ribosylates G_s, activating an adenylate cyclase; ST activates a guanylate cyclase.

20. College student camping through tropical third world country develops abdominal pain and bloody diarrhea. Patient is febrile and liver is enlarged. Diarrhea contains inflammatory cells, cysts, and motile ameboid trophozoites with ingested red cells. Nucleus has a sharp central karyosome. ⑩ CA? Description of the pathology? ↙

   Entamoeba histolytica. The organism is highly invasive and produces flask-shaped ulcers responsible for the characteristic extraintestinal spread.

21. Medical student complains of severe fatigue of 2 weeks' duration and sore throat; physical findings include fever, palpable spleen, postauricular cervical lymphadenopathy, and exudative pharyngitis ⓠ CA? Which antibodies give positive screening test, and what do they cross-react with? ✍

   Epstein-Barr virus. Heterophile antibodies cross-react with animal red cells, not the virus.

22. Febrile neonate born after extended rupture of membranes; mother also febrile. Infant has Apgar scores of 2 and 7 at 1 and 5 minutes, respectively. ⓠ CA? ✍

   Streptococcus agalactiae

Abbreviations

Ac.	*Actinomyces*
ASO	antistreptolysin O (titer)
ATP	adenosine triphosphate
CA	causative agent
cAMP	cyclic adenosine monophosphate
CAMP test	Test that identifies Group B beta-hemolytic streptococci (C A M P are the initials of the developers of this test: Christie, Atkins, and Munch-Petersen. No need to memorize names.)
CF	cystic fibrosis
CIE	counterimmunoelectrophoresis
CNS	central nervous system
CSF	cerebrospinal fluid
DIC	disseminated intravascular coagulation
DR	drug resistance or drug resistant
EA	early antigens
EBNA	Epstein-Barr nuclear antigens
EBV	Epstein-Barr virus
EE	equine encephalitis
EF	edema factor
EHEC	enterohemorrhagic *E. coli*
EIA	electroimmunoassay
EIEC	enteroinvasive *E. coli*
ELISA	enzyme-linked immunosorbent assay
EPEC	enteropathogenic *E. coli*
ETEC	enterotoxic *E. coli*
G+	Gram-positive
G−	Gram-negative
GAS	Group A *Streptococcus*
GBS	Group B *Streptococcus*
GI	gastrointestinal
GU	genitourinary
HSV	herpes simplex virus
HUS	hemolytic uremic syndrome
IL	interleukin
IM	infectious mononucleosis
IV	intravenous
LCM	lymphocytic choriomeningitis

LF	lethal factor
LT	labile toxin (*E. coli* labile toxin)
LTR	long terminal repeat
MAC	membrane activation complex (a.k.a. serum resistance)
MDR	multiple drug resistance (resistant)
MRSA	methicillin resistant *Staphylococcus aureus*
M. tb.	*Mycobacterium tuberculosis*
NA	nucleic acid
NAD	nicotinamide adenine dinucleotide
OMP	outer membrane protein
PAM	primary amebic meningoencephalitis
PBP	penicillin-binding protein
PCR	polymerase chain reaction
PID	pelvic inflammatory disease
PMNs	polymorphonuclear neutrophil leukocytes
PPD	purified protein derivative
pt	patient
RBCs	red blood cells
RES	reticuloendothelial system
R factor	resistance factors
RSV	respiratory syncytial virus
SPE A-C	*Streptococcus pyogenes* erythrogenic toxins A to C
spp	species
STD	sexually transmitted diseases
TB	tuberculosis
TIG	tetanus immune globulin
TNF	tumor necrosis factor
TSS	toxic shock syndrome
TSST-1	toxic shock syndrome toxin
UTI	urinary tract infection
VAPP	vaccine-associated paralytic poliomyelitis
VCA	viral capsid antigen
VTEC	verotoxic *E. coli*
VZV	varicella-zoster virus
WHO	World Health Organization

Index

References in *italics* indicate figures; those followed by "t" denote tables